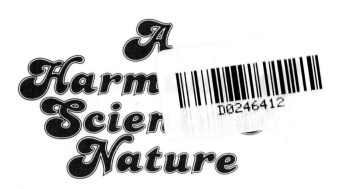

A Harmony of Science & Nature

Ways of Staying Healthy in A Modern World

John & Lucie Davidson

All About:

NATURAL FERTILITY AWARENESS
IRIDOLOGY – NATURAL DIAGNOSIS
WATER POLLUTION & PURIFICATION
JUICE, JUICERS & JUICE EXTRACTION
HEATING PADS & REFLEX FOOT ROLLERS
GRAIN MILLS * WHOLE LIVE MOUSE TRAPS
TIP-U-UP'S AND GRAVITY – PUT YOUR FEET UP
BOWEL CLEANSING THROUGH THE USE OF ENEMAS
PULSORS, SUBTLE ENERGY, & ELECTROMAGNETISM
HERBAL TABLET MAKERS * HERBALISM * CAPSULE FILLERS
CELLULAR STIMULATION THROUGH AEROBIC REBOUNDING
AIR IONIZATION * ELECTROSTATIC FIELD PROTECTION * VDU FILTERS
STAINLESS STEEL STEAMERS * FULL SPECTRUM LIGHTING * LIGHT THERAPY EQUIPMENT
ALLERGY CONTROL PRODUCTS * ALOE VERA MOTHER PLANTS

CONTENTS

CHAPTER 1

YOUR BODY – YOUR LIFE – YOUR CELLS – YOUR PLANET

Our physical body, at the dense physical level, is comprised of millions upon millions of cells. These cells represent a basic unit of physical life. Indeed, the simplest of living creatures that one ever studies in biology classes are single-celled organisms – amoeba, protozoans and their like. When the ovum is fertilized by a sperm, at conception, one cell is formed and from this one cell, through the governing of its chromosomal or genetic material in the nucleus, all other cells are formed by cell growth and division. All normal cells have the same nuclear, chromosomal, genetic or controlling material, but due to factors which are little understood scientifically speaking, as the embryo develops these cells differentiate into particular tissues and organs with differing functions within the body complex, each drawing on what it needs by way of controlling influences, from the relevant parts of the cell nuclei. It seems clear from modern research that there are also subtle, as well as electronic and magnetic energies which play a major part as the energy blueprint from which the body as a whole, its organs and tissues are derived.

Just as plants in a garden can grow strong and healthy or weak and sickly according to the growth and nutritional factors available in their environment, so too do the cells of our body respond to environmental and nutritional factors, growing vibrant with health and well-being or merely struggling to survive from day to day.

In this book, we study some of the factors which influence our level of health and well-being – physical, emotional and mental. While the spiritual life is of paramount importance to us and can be affected by our lower energies and vice versa, that is not our subject in this particular book, but please do not think that we are unaware of it. Indeed, it is only from an understanding of the mystical and spiritual side of life that one can see physical, emotional and mental life in their true perspective.

And so we take a look at nutrition, in the form of pure fruit and vegetable juices and at the effects of pollution in our air, water and electromagnetic environment. We briefly explore the interpenetration of our gross physical being with more subtle energies and we examine how exercise brings strength and nutrition to the cells of our body. We describe a natural solution to the problems of conception and contraception that will not be popular with the drug and contraceptive device companies, but which is a knowledge that all women should possess. And we talk about enemas and the cleansing of the bowels, so that only the sweetest nutrition is absorbed into our body and not the toxins from a lower bowel compost heap.

We look, too, at iridology – a powerful and detailed means of non-invasive, natural diagnosis and we stop briefly to examine back problems and gravity inversion therapy, at ways of making herbs into tablets, at reflexology, at heat treatment, at milling your own cereals and pulses and even at a humane mousetrap that allows you to be free of a forced co-existence with mice without killing them!

A Harmony of Science and Nature, is a survey, with a strong practical bias, because at every step we tell you what items of equipment will be of help to you, available, we have to admit, from our own Wholistic Research Company. But it is quite honest to say that we ourselves use in our own life items from all the product categories available through this company. They all have our personal recommendation. They all help towards a healthy lifestyle in our modern world.

The word **wholistic**, also spelt 'holistic', conveys the idea that the whole is greater than just the sum of its parts. In health, it means considering the 'whole' person – their lifestyle, habits, constitution, physical and emotional strengths and weaknesses. The wholistic minded therapist, practitioner or person therefore considers the whole person, when giving treatment, advice and help. The derivations of 'wholism' and 'holism' are of interest. It seems likely that the word 'holism' was first coined early in this century, having as its root the Greek 'holos' meaning 'whole'. The word 'whole' comes from the old English 'hal', first aquiring a 'wh' in the fifteenth century, and being the same root for 'hale' and 'health'. 'Wholism' was a later variant of 'holism', which gave it a parallel derivation and, in fact, a mildly different flavour of meaning. 'Wholism', is actually 'holism' as applied to health.

We have only ourselves. Whatever we may consider that self to be, it definitely has body and mind wrapped up in it somewhere or somehow. And if that body is not healthy, it is more difficult to be happy and to feel fulfilled. If we spend so much on television sets, motor cars, washing machines, refrigerators and the like, in order to make the running of our lives smoother and more pleasant, then we definitely owe it to ourselves to look after ourselves as well as possible, to give ourselves a better life. In addition, we also have to deal, in some way or another, with the many aspects of environmental pollution and psychological stress engendered by our modern way of life. However, as a friend once commented 'Most people would rather die, than spend £5 a week on their health'. With the current upsurge of interest in Natural Health and the increasing individual desire to take responsibility for one's health and well-being, we hope he is not correct!

So we hope you enjoy this introduction to a wide variety of topics and are stimulated to take your studies more deeply. It is both fascinating and worthwhile – our planet needs care and love if it is to survive as a reasonable place in which to live.

CHAPTER TWO

JUICE, JUICERS AND JUICE EXTRACTION

Juice

Our bodies consist of the food, water and air we consume, organized by life's inner energies and processes into our cells, tissues and organs. It stands to clear reason, therefore, that a healthy body can only be built out of high quality nutrition and pollutant-free foodstuffs. It has always seemed strange to me that people feed themselves on junk foods and low quality produce. Even stranger is the lack of appreciation of true dietary considerations in most medical and hospital practice. How can a person regain good health on hospital canteen food? Yet ask someone to run his car on parrafin, and he will look disbelievingly at you. We need to learn, therefore, what is helpful and what is fad, and what works for us in the maintenance of good health and well being.

It is for this reason, therefore, that the use of fresh fruit and vegetable juices in both normal and therapeutic diets has long been established as a great aid to natural health, energy and well being. The high mineral and nutrient content, combined with the vibrant life-energy of fresh fruits and vegetables, makes pure, fresh juice a wonderful part of a healthy person's diet. In no other way, for example, can one consume the nutritional content of a pound or two of apples and carrots – and then go on to eat a healthy breakfast.

For high quality health, our cells require high quality nutrition. And for this nutrition to be of use, all the tissues and organs of our body must be in prime condition. It is no use, for example, eating excellent healthy food if the epithelial cells lining the intestines are in such poor state that little nutrition is actually absorbed. Nor does it help us if our cardio-vascular or circulatory system is sluggish or the blood is full of uneliminated toxins due to poor kidney, lymph, skin or bowel functioning – the nutrition just never reaches the cells, or is delivered along with unwanted toxins. Similarly, if the lungs do not aerate the blood efficiently or if our muscle tone is weak, we cannot be in good health.

All the cells in our body are in constant change – they grow, they live, they die. Some live for only a few hours, some much longer, but the constant change-over of cells within our body gives us the ability to regenerate healthy tissues by changing our living and eating habits. The existing cells are then strengthened by receiving good nutrition and new cells develop in a more nourishing environment.

Freshly prepared juice contains the subtle life principle, or prana, that energizes our cellular metabolism. It is a powerful vibration interpenetrating the atomic and molecular structure of all the foods we eat. This is why raw fruit and vegetables give us more energy and sparkle than cooked, dead foods. In juice, this energy is concentrated, and you feel it as soon as you drink it. It can clear your head and make you feel light and energetic. It is the presence of this prana, or life energy that writers like Dr. Norman Walker are referring to when they speak of *organic* water and minerals. Water from a tap is 'dead' water, similarly with its mineral content, or table salt, while the water and minerals available in fruit and vegetable juices are already bound into living structures by the synthesing metabolism of the plants. They are full of vibrating life energy, probably discernable even at sub-atomic, if not molecular level.

One may eat a full three cooked meals a day and yet be starved of the basic, vital nutritional elements – the vitamins, enzymes, amino acids, minerals and all the other food requirements destroyed or denatured in the cooking process. We do not say that one should eat only raw fruit and vegetables and their juices, but a balanced healthy diet must contain a good proportion of them.

'Fruit juices are the cleansers of the human system' says Dr. Walker, while 'Vegetable juices are the builders and regenerators of the body.' They contain all the essential nutrients, provided they remain uncooked. Fresh juices are an invaluable supplement to any person's diet, indeed there are therapies that rely almost entirely on the power and nutrition available in juices to rid an ailing body of serious illness, even cancer. The body is stimulated by such concentrated goodness to throw off negative, pathological cellular deterioration and regain excellent health. In a normal regular diet, Dr. Walker recommends the consumption of between two and eight pints per day of fresh juices.

Different fruits and vegetables contain different nutritional elements and there is no doubt that a mixture of juices is of great value. Carrot juice, for example contains all the major vitamins. It helps to promote the appetite and aids digestion. It improves the bone structure of the teeth. The quality of breast milk in nursing mothers is enhanced, while during the last months of pregnancy, Dr. Walker again says that raw carrot juice, taken in sufficient quantities reduces the possibilities of puerperal sepsis at childbirth. 'One pint of carrot juice,' he says, 'has more constructive body value than 25 pounds of calcium tablets.'

The list of benefits of specific juices is extensive and we do recommend Dr. Walker's books, particularly his classic: *Raw Vegetable Juices*. Carrot juice, is a natural solvent for ulcerous and cancerous conditions. It resists infections, working in conjunction with the adrenal glands, including those of the eye, throat, tonsils and sinuses. The nervous system is protected, while vigour and vitality are increased.

Cabbage juice is good for healing duodenal ulcers and constipation and is an excellent source of Vitamin C. Celery juice is high in organic sodium, one property of which is to maintain calcium in solution. It is of great value to people who have used concentrated sugars and starches throughout their lives. It is useful to sufferers from arthritis.

And so the list continues, Dr. Walker and other natural therapists discuss the use of alfalfa, beetroot, coconut, cucumber, brussel sprout, dandelion, endive, fennel, garlic, artichoke, kelp, leek, lettuce, onion, papaya, parsley, parsnip, pepper, potato, radish, rhubarb, sorrel, spinach, tomato, runner bean, turnip, watercress and other juices.

These juices are related to their use in particular conditions from anaemia, allergy, asthma and arthritis to blood pressure, boils, cataracts, colds, chicken pox, cramps, eczema, fatigue, haemorrhoids, hay-fever, headaches, indigestion, insomnia, leukaemia, jaundice, weight control, migrane, nervousness, pregnancy, paralysis, rheumatism, children's diseases, tumours and many other common and uncommon ailments.

Juices are a pure, natural food, full of essential goodness and the body cells respond to them in an energetically positive fashion.

6

Juicers

The concept of relatively inexpensive kitchen juicers, mass produced in plastic and steel or aluminium has become so widely accepted that the quality or quantity of juice produced or the method of extraction is often never questioned. We feel that such juicers mostly pander to a market, at a price that most folk can easily afford, the criterion of marketability being more apparent than that of excellence in juice extraction.

The juicers that we recommend are in a different league and take the matter more seriously. They are, in general, more expensive, but the quality is far superior, both in manufacture and juice content and can genuinely be considered as a part of a naturally healthy lifestyle and an investment in good health.

However, we do not ignore the fact that these inexpensive juicers are widely used and use of the HEALTH STREAM PRESS on the pulp from such juicers can finish off much of what is left undone! We also have a recommendation as to the best of these less expensive juicers.

In order to extract juice from fruits and vegetables, it is necessary to first break down the cell walls and fibres and then separate out the juice. Ideally, a top quality juicer should deliver clear juice on the one hand and a dry pulp of cell walls and fibres, on the other. Generally speaking, commercial and domestic juicers adopt one of three methods to achieve this end.

1. **Centrifugal Juicers** use a grater to more or less break up the plant fibres and cell walls and then spin out the juice by centrifugal action, forcing the pulp against a high speed revolving basket, thrusting the juice through the holes in the basket. This is the least expensive method and hence most domestic juicers follow this design. However, centrifugal juicers suffer from a number of drawbacks:

   (a) The fruit or vegetable is merely grated. At no time is it rubbed or chewed, so the fibres and cell walls are not adequately broken up to allow the extraction of top quality juice. This type of juicer is usually equipped with a tiny, inexpensive high speed motor that would break down completely under a true pulping or mastication process.

   (b) The pulp usually remains very moist, sometimes so moist that considerably more juice can even be squeezed out by hand pressure. The juice itself is pale, watery, low in nutrient value and often quite insipid in flavour.

   (c) The juice is not adequately strained from the cell wall and fibrous material, thus leaving the juice cloudy. With modern methods of agriculture, this can be quite serious. Fruits and vegetables may deposit the non bio-degradable elements of herbicides, insecticides and fertilizers etc. in their cell walls, since they do not have the physiological eliminative channels of higher creatures. That is, once inside, pollutants can't get out. For pure juice, from non-organically grown produce, it is therefore essential to adequately strain the juice under pressure, through a fine mesh juice cloth.

   (d) Enzymes and large molecules are to some extent destroyed by the cutting and centrifugal action, while considerable degrading oxidation of the juice also occurs.

(e) Separate, continuous removal of the pulp is not always possible. It is usually necessary to stop the machine at regular intervals, remove the pulp and start again – a tedious process.

2. **Nose–Cone Pressure Juicers**, such as the CHAMPION and the HEALTH FOUNTAIN, break up the fruit or vegetable material with a cutter or masticator and then ram the resulting pulp into a nose cone with a narrow opening. A high pressure builds up in the cone and the juice is forced out through a stainless steel grid, while the pulp finds its way out through the opening. This is far more efficient than centrifugal action. The power required to efficiently masticate the fruit or vegetable and to build up sufficient pressure in the cone is considerable and the CHAMPION uses a $\frac{1}{3}$ horse-power motor running at 1425 revs per minute. The pressure can also be built up more slowly through the leverage obtained in a manual system, such as the HEALTH FOUNTAIN.

3. **Juice Presses** – and the only available one in the United Kingdom is the HEALTH STREAM JUICER – do the job thoroughly. First, a high powered cutter, such as the CHAMPION, is used to reduce even hard root vegetables to a fine pulp in a few seconds. This is then placed in a strong nylon twill, juice cloth inside a stainless steel pan. A beechwood pressing block is placed on top and the pan and contents placed on the pressing platform. The platform is raised and a pressure of three to five tons is produced between the pressing platform and the top of the press casing. The pulp is pressed flat and the juice, finely strained through the nylon twill cloth, runs out of a spout in the stainless steel pan. The pulp is reduced to something resembling a piece of cardboard, with almost all the juice being pressed out. This method of pulping and then hydraulic pressing is used commercially, on a larger scale, and is generally accepted as the only way to successfully and efficiently extract all the plant juices and nutrients.

Some Facts and Figures
The figures reproduced below from the work of Leroy J Bailey, an independant consultant chemist from Washington, Utah, clearly show the results obtained from the three kinds of juicer in action. 'A' is a centrifugal juicer, 'B' is the CHAMPION and 'C' is a hydraulic press juicer. Apart from the greater quantities of juice produced by the press and the CHAMPION, it is of importance to note that the *concentration* of nutrient and mineral content in the extracted juice *rises* as more juice is extracted. It seems that the last ten percent of juice comes out with a far higher content than the first ten percent. Also, efficient pulping and pressing results in a higher percentage of nutrients being extracted, even if the quantity of juice extracted remains the same. Uniform five pound samples of carrots, celery and parsley were processed by each of the machines with the following results:

	CARROTS			PARSLEY			CELERY		
	A	B	C	A	B	C	A	B	C
Juice extracted – ozs	40.5	47.5	57.0	8.80	10.80	27.0	50.7	69.7	68.1
Mineral Content – mgs									
Calcium as CA	501	1458	2708	460	500	1605	345	505	675
Magnesium as MgO	Tr	5.7	22.8	75	85	265	170	305	385
Phosphorous as P_2O_2	20.3	70.9	285	110	115	445	200	305	480
Iron as FeO	10.5	10.1	37.6	5	10	45	Tr	5	5
Potassium as K_2O	8.1	16.2	31.9	1245	1745	5415	3550	5070	6465
Sodium				100	110	365	1635	1995	2315

The extremely fine pulp produced by a juicer such as the CHAMPION, before processing with the very great pressure of the hydraulic press of machine 'C' would appear to account for the greater yield of juice and the very marked superiority in the extraction of mineral content.

THE VITAMINE CENTRIFUGAL JUICER (A)

We can recommend this juicer as the best centrifugal juicer we have tried. It has many of the drawbacks we describe above, but some juice is definitely better than none and if cost is of prime consideration, then we suggest the VITAMINE as an excellent compromise.

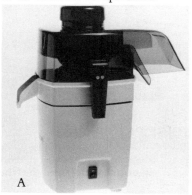

A

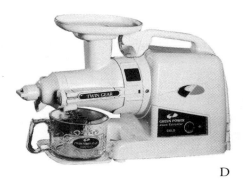

D

The VITAMINE has the following advantages over other centrifugal juicers:

1. The cutting disc and centrifuge basket are made of stainless steel. This is the only centrifugal juicer we know of that does not use aluminium discs and baskets. Aluminium is poisonous. Natural health literature contains many references to this by well qualified and respected naturopathic doctors (Jensen, Walker etc.). It has also been related in conventional medical research to senile dementia, diseases of the nervous system and infant deaths. The VITAMINE's manufacture is of reasonably sturdy plastic and stainless steel, lasting well. It is easy to take apart and clean.

2. The VITAMINE juice extracton capability is superior to other centrifugal juicers that we have tried. With some, you can even extract considerably more juice from the pulp by squeezing it in your hand! Its operation is quick, easy and continuous. It is also automatic in the sense that the pulp is ejected continuously. With many inexpensive centrifugal juicers, you need to make

frequent stops in order to clean the pulp from the basket.

THE CHAMPION JUICER (B)
The CHAMPION is one of the most popular juicers. It is an excellent juicer in its own right, giving an even better performance when used in conjunction with the HEALTH STREAM JUICE PRESS. Using carrots and apples in our tests, we have consistently produced between 25% and 35% more juice by using the CHAMPION as a pulper, and then extracting the juice in our own press. The CHAMPION can also be used for making seed and nut butters as well as soft fruit ice creams and delicious purees. There is also a grain mill available for use with the CHAMPION.

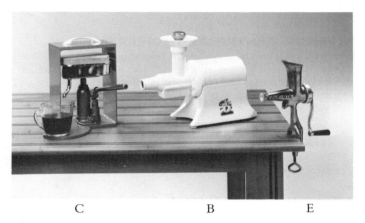

C   B   E

THE HEALTH STREAM MANUAL JUICE PRESS (C)
Using a manually operated three-ton hydraulic ram, the pulp from any juicer that gives a well broken up pulp can be pressed to great advantage, normally giving between 25% and 200% more juice depending on the juicer and the fruit or vegetable being juiced. Normally this press is used along with the CHAMPION, but is also available separately to upgrade the performance of your existing juicer. The Gerson therapists for cancer and other serious illnesses insist on the highest quality juice as an integral part of the therapy. For this purpose, the HEALTH STREAM PRESS is essential. There is also a MOTORIZED HEALTH STREAM which operates at the press of a button.

THE GREEN POWER JUICE EXTRACTOR (D)
The GREEN POWER is a new award-winning juicer from Korea. It is exceptionally good at juicing wheatgrass, herbs and fibrous, leafy greens, and pretty good at carrots, apples, citrus fruit and so on. See separate leaflet for details.

THE HEALTH FOUNTAIN JUICER (E)

The HEALTH FOUNTAIN extracts juice from fruits and vegetables by using a coarse feed screw to cut and propel pieces of fruit and vegetable into a nose cone. The outlet from the nose cone has an adjustable screw to vary the pressure built up in the cone, depending on the fruit or vegetable being juiced. Thus, an almost dry cylinder of pulp comes from the nose cone outlet, while the juice is forced through a stainless steel strainer. For maximum results on hard vegetables such as carrots, the pulp can be reprocessed with a higher pressure.

The system is, or course, slower than the CHAMPION but is considerably less expensive and does produce a high proportion of good quality juice. The HEALTH FOUNTAIN is solidly built, plated, cast iron, somewhat in the style of an old-fashioned mincer. It is not at all beautiful by modern standards unless one described it as 'ruggedly good looking', but it should last a lifetime, outliving many generations of its more modern plastic relatives. We look on it as a specialist wheatgrass and herb juicer, with only occasional use for regular fruits and vegetables.

There is also a less expensive manual juicer, the PORKERT, from the Czech Republic, which works well on wheatgrass and fibrous materials. Built along the lines of an old-fashioned mincer, it is tin-plated, cast-iron and needs care to avoid rusting, but otherwise it works well.

Juicing Wheatgrass and Other Fibrous Plant Life

Wheatgrass juice is used in a number of therapies and being so high in chlorophyll is a valuable addition to a normal healthy diet. Dr. Ann Wigmore, founder of world famous Hippocrates Health Institute in the U.S.A., is the one who really started using wheatgrass juice in therapy and her books are well worth reading. Dr. Jensen's excellent book: 'Health Magic Through Chlorophyll' also describes in detail, the great value of this kind of chlorophyll-rich juice. Chlorophyll is unique in nature. It stands at the base of all food chains. Chlorophyll is the only commonly occuring compound within living organisms able to trap the sun's energy. This same energy is transmitted − through food chains − to all other creatures on this planet. It is similar in molecular structure to the haemoglobin in the blood of all higher animals.

One unique feature of the HEALTH FOUNTAIN is that while the CHAMPION uses a sharp serrated cutting edge, the HEALTH FOUNTAIN uses a coarse screw. This makes it suitable for juicing extremely stringy vegetables such as wheatgrass and comfrey, which otherwise get caught on the serrated cutting edges of other machines. Celery, being both a juicy and stringy vegetable is about as stringy as you can juice with the CHAMPION.

Technical Details (approx)

	Pressure Developed	Motor HP	Revs Per Minute	Weight (lbs)	Height (ins)	Width (ins)	Depth (ins)
HEALTH FOUNTAIN (Manual)	−	−	Manual	5.5	15	3	8
CHAMPION	−	1/3	1425	20	9.3	7.5	18.5
HEALTH STREAM PRESS (Manual)	4 ton	−	−	30	13	8.25	6
HEALTH STREAM PRESS (Motorized)	2–5 tons	−	−	65	16	10	14
GREEN POWER	−	1/4	90	22	15	10	22

CHAPTER THREE

WATER PURIFICATION & POLLUTION –
THE HEALTH VALUE OF DISTILLED WATER

The sections on water pollution and purification are reprinted from 'Water For The Eighties – A Cause For Concern', by Eldon C. Muelhing.

Water Pollution

In virtually all parts of the country, purification procedures are necessary to rid public drinking water of pollutants. Even the simplest 'natural' pollutants – mineral deposits and bacteria, for instance – can accumulate in a water supply, rendering the water either unappetizing or, in some cases, actually hazardous for drinking.

With the introduction of animals or humans to an area, bacterial contamination of water supplies invariably increases because of the animal and human wastes and the decaying garbage that eventually finds its way back into the water.

Agriculture, one of the major users of water, is also one of its major polluters. Fertilizers, pesticides, herbicides and fungicides can be carried off by rain to the nearest water supply, or can seep into the soil eventually contaminating underground well and reservoir sources.

By far the most serious water pollution problems can be attributed to modern industry. Industrial plants often require large volumes of water for production purposes. Most of them are therefore situated near a large body of water for easy access to the quantities they need. However, the close proximity of these water supplies to the industries they serve also makes them a convenient repository for the waste material most industries must discharge as a result of manufacturing processes. In fact, virtually all public and industrial sewage systems are designed to eventually empty into a water supply.

Pollution also occurs closer to our taps than we might realize. Consider the network of pipes that deliver water from a local water treatment plant to a residential area – as well as the plumbing that carries water into a house and its kitchen. The solubility of water allows it to pick up and dissolve particles of a variety of metals with which it might come into contact, such as iron, copper, brass, lead and cadmium. In some areas, worn and outdated water mains have allowed agricultural soil pollutants to seep into the distribution network.

Some people even consider the fluoridation and chlorination of public drinking water a form of contamination. The practice of fluoridation became popular during the 1950's after studies concluded that the natural presence of calcium fluoride in certain water supplies around the country reduced tooth decay. Part of the controversy surrounding fluoridation involves the commonly-used fluoridation additive, sodium fluoride, rather than the naturally occurring calcium fluoride.

Of the many hazards of pollution, the most obvious, of course, is disease caused by bacteria and viruses – microbiological organisms – that contaminate water as a result of human, animal and vegetable sewage deposits.

Certain inorganic substances, found naturally in some water supplies, in plumbing materials, or as a result of industrial wastes, can be harmful to the body in even small amounts. These include such known poisons as arsenic, lead, aluminium, mercury and copper. Other materials, such as calcium, magnesium and iron are among the more common inorganic substances in water and generally account for its 'hardness'. Most of us are familiar with these hard water deposits found at the bottom of kettles or around taps and drains. While such trace minerals have traditionally been considered essential to physical health, some experts now suspect that inorganic minerals from water can accumulate in the body and may be related to certain digestive and kidney problems, arthritis, rheumatism and hardening of the arteries.

The most insidious pollutants, however, are the organic substances which are discharged in the form of detergents, pesticides, petroleum or other hydrocarbons – chemical substances which do not dissolve in water, but which can interact in water with one another, or with inorganic substances, to form entirely new chemicals. For example, chlorine (inorganic) can react with decomposing leaves (organic) to create the toxic compound chloroform. Because of the vast number of organic compounds being developed annually – as many as five hundred new substances are introduced each year – the possible reaction combinations are multiplying astronomically. In many cases neither the results nor the effects of these potential combinations have been determined.

Organic pollutants in water can have another serious effect, attracting 'decomposer bacteria' which utilize the oxygen in water, thus suffocating and eventually killing off entire populations of fish. The shorelines of polluted lakes and rivers cease to be attractive to residential and resort developers, and untreated pollutants can render water unusable for irrigation or other agricultural purposes.

The thermal pollution of water can also have adverse effects on the environment. Thermal pollution is actually nothing more than heated water which has been used as a coolant for certain industrial processes and then put back into the water supply: for example, water that has been used to cool a steam-powered generator. Increasing the natural temperature of a water supply even a few degrees, however, can interrupt the delicate environmental balance in vegetation and wildlife which are susceptible to sudden variations and changes in temperature.

A less prevalent but still existent form of water pollution is the presence of harmful radioactive substances which can be introduced into a water supply as a result of the mining or processing of radioactive materials, waste from nuclear power plants or fallout from nuclear testing.

Domestic Water Pollution

Many of us do not stop to think where all the life-destroying chemicals in the detergents and cleaning fluids that we pour down our sinks, toilets and drains actually end up. They are mostly undestroyable or they recombine with other substances that they come across and are generally toxic to life. Can you imagine how many *millions of tons* of poisonous materials per year come from our own homes and are ultimately emptied into rivers and the sea? And how this water and its pollutants finds its way into reservoirs and back into our tap water, as well as into our food? This is why it is important to use bio-degradable products as much as possible.

Historians of the future will probably call our century, the 'Plastic Age' or the 'Dirty Century' and look with extreme disfavour upon the legacy of destruction we have left them. Perhaps there was no other way to 'advance' technologically, but isn't it time we gave top priority to cleaning up the mess in our own backyard, before it submerges us completely? It is only selfish interests and ignorance that prevent this happening.

We may think, naively, that perhaps 'they' (government? industry? United Nations?) would tell us of dangers in our water and environment (if 'they' knew!). But 'they', in fact, are ourselves and all of us are constrained by so many factors, as well as prejudice and lack of knowledge, that the issues have become unclear. So much money is spent, for example, on road safety, yet thousands more people die of cigarette smoking than on the roads, a problem that could be solved by simply making it illegal to sell tobacco. But the ramifications of such a move are immense – the loss of jobs and livelihood, the interplay of international relationships with tobacco growing countries, the loss of taxation revenue, the loss of votes. It needs to be done, but what politician is man enough (or woman enough) to put his (or her) neck on the block to even formulate a phasing out of the tobacco industry?

So with problems of such magnitude facing us, what chance do the relatively under-researched effects of water pollution have of being dealt with? Ultimately it becomes a personal decision. The only problem, of course, is getting hold of the right facts upon which to base a decision.

Water Purification

While the pre-treatment of public water before it is made accessible for drinking has been widely practiced for more than a century, post-treatment of 'used' water before it reenters the water supply is relatively new. Methods of combating pollution at its source have been developed and used successfully in the treatment of public sewage and industrial waste water. However, in many cases, the money as well as the technological knowledge required to treat certain of the new pollutants is still lacking.

While all of us acknowledge the need for strict public regulation to maintain safe water supplies, some critics of the specific quality standards, as set forth by the government and World Health Organization etc., note that they are too lenient on the one hand and too stringent on the other. In other words, they claim, water should be treated according to the way in which it is going to be used. Must the water used to fight fires undergo the same expensive cleansing procedures as the water we drink? And what of the water we drink? Are the results of the costly treatment at the local treatment site negated as the water passes through the worn and outdated water mains that pipe it to our homes? If treatment facilities are to be upgraded, shouldn't the entire water distribution networks in our cities and towns be upgraded too?

These questions posed by the critics are, of course, expensive ones. Two grades of water – or perhaps ideally three: a utility grade for fire-fighting, watering lawns and flushing toilets; a work grade for household uses such as bathing and washing clothes; and, a third grade for drinking and cooking would require untold amounts of money if the three were to be piped separately to the general public from the water company.

Nor would the up-grading of water mains ensure the purity of our tap water unless we replaced outdated plumbing systems in our individual homes as well. New and different approaches to solving the water pollution problem are presented almost daily, but the cost and practicality of many preclude their implementation on a large scale.

The government is not the only one attempting to develop solutions, however. The private sector of society has made significant inroads, most notably in the area of improving drinking water quality as it comes out of our taps. In the past few decades a number of water purification techniques, designed for use in the home, have been developed and perfected. In addition, bottled water has made a come-back in areas where pollution problems have been widely publicized. Bottled water, however, can vary almost radically in quality. To date there are no uniform regulations governing the quality of domestic bottled water. Even those labelled as natural mountain or natural spring water have been subjected to a variety of natural pollutants and are treated in some way prior to bottling. The manufacturers cannot simply put a bottle to the hillside spring and then cork it up!

Other alternatives to drinking ordinary tap water have become so popular so fast that most of us are unfamiliar with both the processes themselves and with the expected results.

Following are just some of the items a one might encounter when shopping for a home water purification or treatment system.

Water Softeners remove hardness – minerals such as calcium and magnesium – and replace them with sodium through a process of ion-exchange. This artificially softens the water making it more effective for washing clothes or dishes and bathing. Because of the increased sodium content, this water is not recommended for drinking, particularly for individuals on a salt restricted diet. In fact, recent medical research points to a more than strong indication that too much salt causes heart disease. Natural medicine has always, of course, warned against the use of too much salt in one's diet.

Filters can remove selected contaminants from water, employing such materials as a screen, a net, porous paper, but most commonly, activated charcoal (charcoal that will attract particles from the water until it is saturated). Charcoal filters generally remove certain dissolved gases, some light organic compounds and can improve the colour of water. They do not, however, affect most dissolved solids, minerals, inorganic ions like nitrates, or bacteria. Water passed through any of the generally available filters is likely to suffer from a variety of problems, the worst of which is bacterial contamination. Filters, as well as reverse osmosis membranes are easily colonized by bacteria which recontaminate the water as it is produced. A high level of supervision is needed to avoid this kind of problem, a supervision more or less impossible in a domestic environment with no adequate means of testing the water. Even if some of the bacteria are filtered out and die, the breakdown of dead micro-organisms can result in such products as pyrogens. Pyrogens are a little understood group of compounds which increase the body temperature if introduced into the blood stream. It is for this reason that distillation remains the sole permitted method for preparing water to be used for injections.

De-Ionizers use an ion-exchange resin to remove mineral ions – electrically charged molecules. Organic materials and molecules, plus suspended and colloidal particles are not removed and some kind of filtration is also required.

Reverse Osmosis Units effectively condition water by separating it from dissolved minerals and chemicals using a semi-permeable membrane, usually manufactured from an organic substance similar to cellophane. The process is not generally as effective in de-mineralizing water as is the de-ionization process, nor does it remove all the micro-biological impurities.

Ultra Filters employ membranes similar to those used in reverse osmosis units, but the method of operation is quite different. The membrane is designed to collect relatively large organic molecules as the water passes through it, but it does not appreciably remove dissolved inorganic solids nor bacteria.

Ultraviolet Purifiers kill bacteria as water runs through a tube, but will not remove other pollutants unless combined with a filtration method.

Bacteriostatic Units are usually used in combination with charcoal filters and suppress the growth of bacteria using ultraviolet rays, chlorine, iodine, or silver.

Chlorinators are designed to kill bacteria with chlorine, but can leave an objectionable taste and odor and can form potentially dangerous chemical compounds. Chlorine, in itself, is a killer to all forms of life and not exactly a welcome addition to our drinking water!

Iodinators purify water with a bed of iodine that works more slowly than chlorine to kill bacteria.

Ozonators use a highly activated form of oxygen to burn up bacteria.

Microstrainers remove bacteria and some chemicals from water, but do not remove nitrates.

Electrodialysis Units demineralize water by passing a current of electricity through it to remove inorganic minerals. This method does not effectively remove organic substances nor bacteria.

Water Distillers simulate the natural hydrologic cycle by boiling water to kill bacteria. As water is vaporized, chemicals and minerals are left behind in the vaporizing chamber. The steam is then condensed in a sterile condensation chamber. While other purification methods must frequently be combined to ensure effectiveness, a distiller is self-contained and usually considered the most effective of water purification processes, producing virtually pure water.

Although de-ionized water is available at chemists, it is not the same as distilled water. As mentioned above, because of potential contamination by bacterial colonization or the breakdown of decomposing micro-organisms, distillation remains the sole permitted method for preparing water to be used for injections. Distllation not only removes them, but it delivers sterile water at 100°C. Moreover, de-ionized water is normally stored in plastic containers, which may also contaminate the water. It is also expensive when used over a period of time, and it becomes cheaper and easier to distill ones's own water at home.

Water Purification Plants

Most of the country's treatment facilities are no longer well-equipped to perform these procedures, having been constructed soon after the processes became established in the 1920's and '30's. Today, many of these treatment procedures and the facilities themselves are considered inadequate for satisfactorily treating the types of agricultural and industrial pollutants that now exist. They are also largely in need of massive renovation.

Britain's Water Supplies

The privatization of the regional Water Authorities in England and Wales, together with our entry into the EEC, has highlighted many of the problems facing Britain's water Industry. In Scotland, water and sewage are still run by the local councils, while in Northern Ireland, they are run directly by the government. This means that while the privatized companies have at least been able to raise some capital for investment in much-needed repair work and modernization programmes, Scotland and Northern Ireland are still dependent upon government hand-outs. They therefore stand in line with hospitals, social services and all other demands upon the public purse. And since politicians tend to make decisions based on where the votes lie, water purity remains low on the list. As they say, "There are no votes in sewage."

The water industry values its assets at about £50 billion. This makes giant national enterprises like British Rail and the National Coal Board pale by comparison. But despite these considerable assets, the sale of the water companies in 1990 was not easy, due to the dreadful condition of the water mains and sewers, as well as the water purification and sewage disposal systems.

The reasons for this are simple: since the 1970s, the government had halved investment in the water industry, leaving it with a massive repair bill and an even more massive bill for modernization to meet today's ecological standards. At the present time, millions of people receive water that is in breach of EEC regulations, in one respect or another. Indeed, in June 1991, the European Commission announced that it intended to prosecute Britain over the illegal levels of pesticide in the drinking water supplied to 10 million people.

This action by the Commission resulted from the Government's failure to force six out of the ten major water companies to meet the European standards. Andrew Lees, Friends of the Earth campaign director, pointed out, "The Government has helped some water companies avoid investment in new treatment plants by allowing them to continue supplying tap water containing illegal levels of pesticide." Though the water companies are reporting high levels of profit, their customers are still receiving tap water which is hazardous to health.

Under the EC Drinking Water Directive, member states had pledged to meet certain pesticide limits by 1985. But in the run-up to privatization, and in their desire to make the sale successful, the Government compromised the health of the nation by permitting more than half of the water authorities to continue supplying contaminated water for up to 15 years beyond the EC deadline. Thames was given until the year 2000, Wessex until 1999, Southern until 1998, Severn-Trent until 1997, Anglian until 1995 and Yorkshire until December 1991.

The worst-hit areas for pesticide pollution include most of the South-East, London, much of East Anglia and the Midlands, parts of western England and Yorkshire, and large areas of Wales. In many cases, levels 20 times higher than those permitted are commonly found. Recent water samples from Thames, showed the levels of five pesticides to be between 6 and 16 times the European limit. Wessex Water has recorded levels of atrazine 21 times over the top, Southern Water samples had eight pesticides up to 10 times the EC limit, Yorkshire had atrazine levels at 5 times the limit and Severn-Trent and Anglian Water had no figures available at all.

Rather than apply greater pressure to the water companies, the British Government's main effort in solving the problem has been an attempt to have the permitted levels of many toxic substances increased. But further EC medical research collaboration has resisted all such attempts. In fact, there is considerable evidence that even the present EC limits are still unsafe, but since there are many European countries in the same predicament as the UK, there is considerable pressure to at least leave them as they are.

Pesticide levels are presently set at 0.1 microgrammes per litre – for any pesticide – a tacit admission that the affects of different pesticides upon health are little understood. It is only known that they are very bad for you, many of them being carcinogenic. And with 1 in 4 people, or some statistics say 1 in 3, likely to develop a cancer during the course of their life – a statistic quite undreamt of in the earlier part of this century – the obvious cause is the widespread ingestion of pollutants from our food, air and water.

The situation regarding other serious pollutants is very similar. Nitrates are a problem in all parts of the country and are still above EC permitted levels. The large agricultural area of East Anglia, mostly served by Anglian Water, has only two nitrate removal plants commissioned at the present time. And when one realizes that each plant can serve a maximum of only 20,000 people, the problem is further highlighted. In fact, these plants are portable – they can be taken from place to place wherever the problem is worst, at any time. So water quality tested one day, could be radically worse on the next, as the plant is moved from place to place.

Iron, manganese and aluminium in the water are also serious contaminants, and the water in many areas is once again above EC permitted limits. In fact, aluminium, as aluminium sulphate, is actually *added* to water in many water treatment works as a coagulent, to remove small particles, even though aluminium has been positively identified by medical research to be implicated in the degeneration of the brain and nervous system, leading to such conditions as Alzheimer's disease (senile dementia) and Parkinson's disease. Aluminium in certain baby foods is also thought to be responsible for some infant cot deaths, and concern has been focussed upon the water supply as another source of toxicity. Aluminium sulphate is particularly used in areas where the water runs through peat and moorland, to remove peat residues from the water – Yorkshire, northern England, Scotland, Wales and Devon being the worst affected.

When dealing with toxic water 'purifiers', mistakes and accidents are also bound to happen from time to time. And by the time the error has been detected and a warning made public, it is usually too late. In the case of the Camelford disaster of 1988, when an engineer mistakenly added a large quantity of aluminium sulphate to the water, large numbers of people were taken seriously ill, many of whom may never fully recover.

Other sources of pollution are the water mains themselves. Some areas of Scotland and the north still have many properties served by lead or lead-lined water mains, long after it has been established that lead is extremely toxic, causing – amongst other things – permanent brain damage to children. And in many areas, the old and antiquated iron pipes are so corroded that blisters account for more than half of their original diameter. In some areas, as much as 50% of the water put into the pipes leaks away into the ground, due to corrosion damage. This was the condition in Liverpool, prior to privatization, and it is likely to be worse by now. It is clear that such a situation is going to take many years to rectify. Towns like Derby, Leicester and Birmingham are the worst hit because of their acid waters. Such advanced corrosion and internal damage to the water mains also results in rust fragments in the tap water (which can rupture reverse osmosis membranes), as well as infestations of small animals and bacteria, the blisters providing ideal homes and breeding grounds. *Nais* worms have also been reported in Sussex and other water supplies. Back in the early 1980s, 20,000 tons of extraneous matter were reported to lie with the water mains of the old *Anglian Water Authority*, about 4 kilos per customer. When it told the House of Lords that it needed an increase in capital investment of 300%, it received a mere 2%. Now, Anglian Water are slowly replacing their 20,000 miles of water mains with flexible, blue plastic pipes, at a cost of one billion pounds. But it will take 15 years to complete.

On first thought, sewage disposal may seem disconnected from tap water supply, but this is not so. Ultimately, all the waste water that flows from our homes ends up in the same rivers, lakes and streams from which our drinking water is derived. Nature shows no selection between the sources of her water; it is all mixed together. And all our household wastes – billions of tons of toxic detergents, disinfectants, soaps, sewage and everything else – get dumped into the planetary water supply when they leave our homes. Some raw sewage is dumped directly into the sea or rivers causing ecological problems of mammoth proportions, while other sewage is cleaned up as best they may. But one can imagine the technical problems involved, many of which remain insurmountable.

And like the water mains, the country's sewage systems are in a dreadful state of repair, suffering from high levels of corrosion. Not so long ago, the North West Water Authority – as it then was – reported 600 major sewage collapses per year (just under two a day), and water mains of which 40% suffered "from an unacceptable degree of corrosion and internal deposits." And Yorkshire made the amazing admission that it knew the whereabouts of only 70% of its sewage system, and the condition of a mere 5%!

This kind of situation is clearly going to require considerable time and expenditure to remedy. Indeed, it now seems an almost impossible task to deliver pure water to our taps. The onus, therefore, falls on the individual to solve the problem within his own home. With the increasing numbers of known and unknown pollutants, we are left with the unavoidable solution of needing to separate pure H_2O from the unknown nasties. For this reason, we personally use and recommend domestic water distillation as the only sure way of dealing with the problem.

Health Value of Distilled Water
Eminent physicians for many years have recognized and advocated the health value of distilled water, both for the prevention of disease and for the restoration of health. C.W. De Lacy Evans, M.D., in his book, 'How To Prolong Life', claims that distilled water, used regularly in place of spring water or other water containing inorganic minerals, tends to ward off the ageing process by preventing the formation of calcareous deposits that cause hardening of the arteries. He writes: 'Used as a drink, distilled water is absorbed directly into the

blood, the solvent properties of which it increases to such an extent that it will keep in solution salts already existing in the blood, prevent their undue deposit in various organs and structures, favour their elimination by the various excreta, and tend to remove these earthy compounds which have already accumulated in the body ... There is no doubt as to the high value of distilled water used freely as a retarder of the ossifying conditions which appear to constitute the condition of old age'.

Occasionally, you find writers who feel that distilled water will remove valuable minerals from the body. This is neither true, nor is it borne out by the evidence from users of distilled water. The concentration of minerals in tap water is very small compared to that in fruits and vegetables and of very little importance to anyone eating a healthy diet. There is so much pollution in our modern times, that distillation is the only way to be sure and be independent of what 'big brother' might do.

Dr. Charles McFerrin, writing in July 1955 issue of 'Nature's Path', writes: 'Distilled water is 'empty' water – a hungry water, a water capable of absorbing body poisons. You may have had the experience of trying to use an old post office blotter on the desk. Everybody has used it and it is so full of ink that it will not suck up any more. So it is with a 'full' water, a water full of chlorine, aluminium, etc. Such water does not have the capacity of absorbing body impurities'. Dr Christopher compares drinking tap water to putting coffee (with milk and sugar) into your car battery.

Free daily use of distilled water is a marvellous blood purifier, helping to bring into solution and dilute any toxins in the body, as well as aid in their elimination through the kidneys. It should be used for cooking and baking as well as for drinking. For health's sake it is important to use only distilled water, which is a supreme internal body-cleansing agent. It aids in the removal of waste matter by bringing into solution and washing out through the excretory channels impurities that have accumulated and settled in the body, such as uric acid deposits that cause rheumatism. It helps promote osmotic interchange through the kidney tubules, thereby furthering the elimination of toxins through the urine.

Distilled water should be stored in glass (not plastic) flagons or bottles and can be energized by keeping the bottles in natural sunlight. If held in coloured glass containers, it can also be utilized in colour therapy. The regular use of distilled water for washing the face and hands, in conjunction with its use in diet and drinking, aids in the creation of a clear, glowing complexion.

Referring to the origin and means of preventing the formation of calcareous deposits in the body, which produce the symptoms of senility by gradually ossifying it, and which come from use of hard water, Dr. de la Torre writes: 'Instead of drinking the hard water of springs or the chlorinated water of the cities, it will be to our advantage to drink distilled water . . . to prevent calcification of the body'.

It is generally admitted by those who have studied the subject that the abundant use of distilled water will help keep the body cells free from accumulated waste products, and thus help to preserve health and prolong life. We are literally 'as old as our arteries', and since ordinary hard water causes the arteries to harden by the deposit of inorganic lime compounds along their inner walls, so, by use of distilled water, which prevents such deposits, the arteries are preserved in a more youthful condition.

Dr. Alexander Graham Bell, inventor of the telephone, recognized the health value of distilled water, and claimed that its daily use prolonged his life. He possessed a water still and made his own. He wrote: 'Some years ago I was afflicted with sciatica, and was bed-ridden on account of it. The doctors could not find anything to relieve me. The attack came just as I was investigating certain subjects relating to the deposit of salts. One was the deposit of salts in the human system. A well known scientist had written a book in which he said that old age came from such deposits, and that the ills of advanced years were due to the lack of their elimination. This man thought that when such deposits went to the joints, man had rheumatism. When they went to the kidneys, he had kidney trouble and stones in the urinary organs: and when they lodged in the arteries, they produced what is called hardening of the arteries. In the same way, when such deposits coated the nerves, they produced sciatica . . . I knew that distilled water was pure. I thought that if I drank plenty of it, I could get rid of some of the salts that were covering my sciatic nerves. I tried drinking it, and it worked like a charm . . . I have kept up my drinking of distilled water and I attribute my almost perfect health largely to it. I have a little still with which I make what I need'.

The **Wholistic Research Company** can supply a full range of water distillers, from small, camping and domestic units, through large and small family distillers, to systems for large health centres where distilled (and even chilled) water can be pumped to locations around the centre. As usual, please request full product information from them.

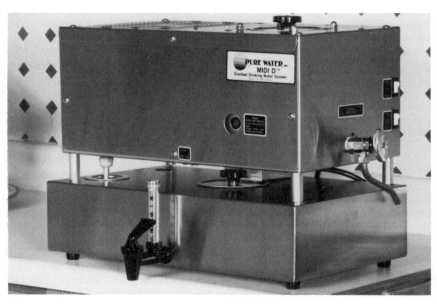

The MIDI-STILL D AUTO – The Best Selling Family Distiller.

CHAPTER FOUR

AIR IONIZATION, THE ATMOSPHERE & BIOELECTRICITY

During this period of the earth's history, when man is spreading his influence into its every corner, it is unfortunately discovered with increasing frequency that this influence has caused an imbalance in nature, harmful to the world eco-system as a whole and in many cases directly harmful to man himself.

With people's short-term interests at stake, or simply because of the pressure of events in daily life, the signs are often ignored or rationalized, building up the problem for future decades and generations.

The quality of the air we breathe is one such problem area. Who has not gone out for a 'breath of fresh air'? – feeling relieved from the stuffiness of an overheated or overcrowded room. Why does an air-conditioned atmosphere feel 'dead'? Why does mountain or sea air make us feel so good and even promote healing? Why does the weather affect our mood? One of the answers lies in the electrical state of the air – in its ionization And the solution – other than living by the sea or in the mountains - can lie in an air ionizer.

Ions are gas molecules that carry an electrical charge, by gaining or losing an electron. In nature they are generated by ultra-violet light from the sun, by lightning and thunderstorms, by background radio-activity in rocks and soil, and by the breaking of water into droplets by waves, waterfalls and mountain streams. Plants, too, are one of nature's most prolific source of negative ions. They conduct the negative electrical charge of the earth up into the air and 'eject' it from the tips of their leaves.

Much research and experimentation has been made. One of the first studies in this century was made by Albert Einstein, who in 1910 – along with a colleague Conrad Harbicht – took as a Ph.D. thesis the problem of why the mountain air of Davos was renowned for its health giving properties. They decided it was 'Air Electricity'. Einstein went on to consider other matters, but Harbicht later got funding to continue his research and the first ionizers were built. It would seem that air ionization – and in particular, negative air ionization – plays an important role in the natural economy.

Negative ions are one of nature's natural sweepers – they aid in the destruction of airborne bacteria by oxidative action and clear dust, pollen, smoke and small particles from the atmosphere. In the body, negative ions increase our capacity to take up oxygen and enhance the ability of the respiratory tract to deal with airborne particles – allergens, dust, smoke etc. Histamine, which triggers hay fever, is reduced in level by negative ions which also have a beneficial effect on anyone suffering from bronchial complaints such as bronchitis, asthma, catarrh and the common cold.

Empirical research has also shown that sufferers of insomnia, migraine, emphysema, eczema, headaches, tiredness, depression and a general feeling of malaise are often helped by an artificially induced increase in the level of negative ions. Hospital burn units, especially in the U.S.A., use negative ion generators in close proximity to the burnt area, and report a widespread increase in the speed and quality of healing.

It is not only man that is affected by the level of ionization. As long ago as 1748, the Frenchman L'Abbe Nollet found that plants placed under charged electrodes grew faster and in 1775, Father Gian Battista Buccaira of the University of Turin, Italy, wrote: 'It appears manifest that nature makes extensive use of atmospheric electricity for promoting vegetation'. Scientists at the University of California grew barley, oats, lettuce and peas in an atomsphere drastically reduced in ionization and found that growth was stunted and the plants diseased. The same experiment in air with more than double the natural number of ions produced accelerated growth. In Russia, scientists tried to raise small animals – mice, rats, guinea pigs, rabbits – in air with no ions in it at all. They all died within a few days.

It seems clear that man and all creatures developed in an ionized atmosphere and while a depletion of this level causes harm, an increase appears to create nothing but good.

In our modern life, we have created an environment that virtually eliminates negative ions from the atmosphere. Pollution from car exhausts, air conditioning, cigarette smoking, overcrowding and even breathing all contribute to this. In addition, fluorescent lighting, electrical and electronic equipment, air conditioning units and static-producing man-made fibres in carpets, clothes and curtains all reduce the level of negative ions and increase the positive.

Offices and organizations that have installed negative ionization equipment have found that their employees are less likely to get colds, report absent less frequently and are generally more cheerful and alert. Submarines and spacecraft scientists have also recommended the use of negative air ionizers in such closed and artificial atmospheres.

In 1969, Dr. Felix Sulman, head of the Applied Pharmacology department at Jerusalem University, found that 'normal' people – his subjects were two groups of men and women between twenty and sixty five – became irritable and fatigued when left for an hour or so in a room that contained a heavy overdose of positive ions. Yet the same people confined for the same period in air containing an overdose of negative ions, showed, via the electroencephalogram, a slower, stronger pulse rate of Alpha waves of the brain than when they were in normal air. (Alpha wave rhythms are considered a measure of the brain's activity and health: A slow, firm pulse rate is generally regarded as an indication of health and increased alertness). He tested their alertness and work capacity by various means and all of them scored significantly higher during and immediately after exposure to a high level of negative ions than in 'normal' air.

In certain areas of the world, there are winds known even through legend as 'evil' or 'witches' winds. These winds all have one factor in common – a high level of positive ionization. Domestic quarrels, suicides, crime rate, traffic accidents and even plane crashes are all blamed on the wind. The Foehn of Southern Europe is one such wind. In one hospital, all operations except emergencies are postponed when the Foehn is blowing, because the incidence of: 'The operation was a success, but the patient died', is that much higher. In the Middle East, some courts even permit the fact that the Sharav was blowing when a crime was committed, to be entered as a plea of mitigation, while in parts of Switzerland and Italy, judges are often known to be lenient if the Foehn was blowing at the time when certain offences were committed. Psychiatrists also have reported a significant increase in urgent calls from their patients at times when these winds blow.

Bioelectricity

Air ionization is another *bioelectrical* phenomenon, discussed briefly in the next chapter. Basically, modern research shows that the body has a complex energy field at the electromagnetic level that affects all aspects of our health and well being – both physiological as well as emotional and mental. There is a direct energy pathway between our inner emotional and mental energies and our physiological – cellular and molecular – processes. Negative air ironization seems to stimulate and balance this energy field, while positive air ionization depresses and disharmonizes it, making us feel tired, depressed and emotional or exhibiting physical problems – aches and pains, changes in blood pressure and so on. These *electrical* aspects of climate are discussed more thoroughly in the next chapter and in the much expanded version in my book, *Subtle Energy*, published in 1987.

It is surprising that we do not give more attention to the air we breathe. We cannot see what is happening to it in our homes and offices and therefore assume that all is fine. Unfortunately, it is not. However, there is a remedy, which lies in the use of negative air ionizers. Models are available for homes, offices, factories, air conditioning systems and the results of their use have often proved quite dramatic.

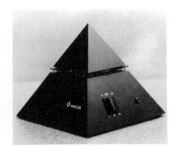

MODULION 10

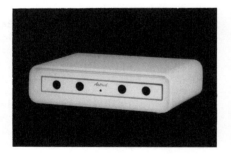

ASTRID

Two of the range of tested ionizers available from the Wholistic Research Company.

Schumann Waves and Electrostatic Field Simulators

As we have pointed out, we live in an environment in which natural electrical and magnetic phenomena have a considerable role to play. Between the ionosphere and the earth's surface, there is a voltage gradient of about 200,000 volts of static electricity representing a differential of about 400 volts between your head and your feet when standing outside in the open air. This electrostatic field is not constant, but varies, containing within it vertical oscillating waves of a fundamental, basic frequency, modulated with many harmonics, the whole having a sequence repeating several times per second. These harmonics extend into the megahertz range and have a regulating and stabilizing influence on physiological processes.

These Schumann waves, as they are called, are a natural part of our environment that are blocked or reduced by many modern building materials and urban environments. Furthermore, for Schumann wave formation, a reasonable level of conductivity is required on the earth's surface. This conductivity relates to the ground water level which in recent times has been reduced through use in industrial applications. Thus, cities, for example, are places of low or absent Schumann wave activity.

In healthy people, the absence of Schumann waves can be tolerated, but in sick people, there is greater need of their stabilizing effect. The absence of Schumann waves is also felt by those under stress and Schumann wave generators are one of the devices used by NASA to keep their astronauts in good psychological and psychological condition.

Also permeating our natural environment is the lithosphere – the earth's magnetic field modulated by electron–plasma waves and ultra-fine energies emitted by trace elements. The Indumed equipment employs magnetic field generators that use iron filament impregnated with these trace elements. The result, along with other refinements to further mimic the natural electron-plasma and Schumann waves, is an instrument that has considerable power as a therapeutic aid across the whole range of human health problems. The research shows that different bodily conditions have different rates or harmonic frequencies, and thus the Indumed instrument has different settings for various conditions. All of this correlates very well, of course, with the findings of radionics which identifies specific vibrational rates with particular organs, diseases and conditions. Some psychics, too, are well aware that different organs, physiological and anatomical, systems and conditions have specific colours as perceived by their subtle sight.

Treatment time using Indumed is about fifteen to thirty minutes per session, but if the Indumed output is fed into the patient after combination with output from a Mora therapy instrument, which is naturally tuned to a patients' individual energies, then not only is the treatment enhanced, but it then takes only three or four minutes to produce the same effect. *In other words, the closer we get to harmonizing the individual's natural energy vibrations within, then the less energy we need to create a deeper and more pronounced an effect.* Mora therapy uses highly sophisticated modern equipment to read in the individual electromagnetic emanations of a patient through the acupuncture points. This energy pattern is then 'cleaned up' electronically, and fed back to the patient, again through the acupunture points.

Magnetic Field Therapy

The use of simple magnets for their therapeutic qualities has long been a part of natural medicine. In modern times, the therapeutic benefits of magnetic field therapy are the subject of on-going research. Since 1974, more that 23 universities and 350 scientists have worked in this field, successfully treating patients with inflammations, rheumatism, pain of many kinds (headaches, migraine, back pain etc.), sleeplessness, poor blood circulation, cancer and various other problems. The most effective forms of treatment combine the three main forms of natural electromagnetic field. These are (i) the electrostatic Schumann waves, (ii) the geomagnetic lithospheric vibrations caused by the presence of trace elements in the earth's crust, and (iii) solar energies in the microwave region of the electromagnetic spectrum. Even brief exposure to these fields can help to stabilize a person's physiology and psychology for some days.

A number of different forms of magnetic therapy are available. Naturally-ocurring magnetic rocks, for example, such as magnetite or lodestone can have some beneficial effects since they contain trace elements, even though they do not recreate the Schumann or solar electromagnetic vibrations. Artificial iron magnets, however, of the kind which are normally available, sometimes in bangles or belts, may have a very limited value above that of a placebo, due to the absence of trace elements.

Two small devices which mimic all three forms of electromagnetic field are MEDISEND and MEDICUR, which are based on the research of German biophysicist, Dr Wolfgang Ludwig. Among Ludwig's many contributions has been a technique for storing the effect of trace elements in magnetic materials by inducing permanent changes in the atomic lattice. He also discovered that Schumann waves alone could have negative side effects, needing to be used in combination with the other two forms of natural electromagnetism.

A form of magnetic material which is impregnated with trace elements, and is hence far more effective than simple magnets alone, is ENERGON magnetic foil. ENERGON comes in two-inch wide strips with the magnetic polarity across the thickness of the material, making application easier and penetration of body tissues much deeper.

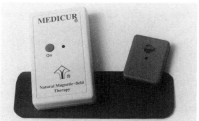

MEDICUR, MEDISEND and ENERGON MAGNETIC FOIL

Magnetic fields effect living tissues in a variety of ways. Since electromagnetism is the force which holds atoms and molecules together in a dynamic interplay and organized interaction, all cellular and bodily processes will be effected to a greater or lesser extent by the presence of these fields. Oxygen molecules, for example, have paramagnetic properties and cells are readily induced to take up more oxygen in the presence of a magnetic field. Pulsed or changing electromagnetic fields give rise to tiny electrical currents in the conductive materials of the body, inducing the movement of electrically-charged molecules within cells. This is a part of the body's natural means of moving substances about and of passing signals throughout the body, as in nerve cells. By judicious use of magnetic fields, magnetically active substances within the body can also be moved from place to place, like iron filings by a magnet.

There are also many indications that link electromagnetic fields to more subtle energies of mind and body, many being discussed in the book *Subtle Energy*. Modern science is slowly moving towards the vibrational and the subtle.

CHAPTER FIVE

PULSORS★, SUBTLE ENERGY & ELECTROMAGNETISM

Excerpts from the Book: Subtle Energy by John Davidson

SUBTLE ENERGY PATHWAYS AND POLARITIES

Modern man is by now well acquainted with the fact that the physical universe as perceived by our five senses is very different in appearance to that which is described by science. This scientific description has changed and is continually changing.

Other species inhabiting this planet have senses which we do not, in their perception of physical matter: some birds have a sense which perceives the magnetic grid of the earth and they use it for migration. Other creatures perceive wavelengths and frequencies of sound and electromagnetic energy (e.g. light) that we cannot. Dogs, horses and other animals seem to have a "sixth sense" – they are aware of the subtle energy vibrations of humans and their fellow creatures. In fact, if we compare the full electromagnetic energy spectrum to a distance of 10,000 miles (Cambridge to Peking), then the range of visible wavelengths, which we call light, and perceive through our eyes, measures a distance of a mere six feet!

Furthermore, even amongst humans, we differ in both our perceptive abilities and in our interpretation of the perceived data! Some people have a far higher frequency range in their hearing than others. Some are colour-blind, an artist sees colours more vividly, musicians may have "perfect pitch", some have altogether lost one or more of their senses, an increasing number are tuned to the subtle vibrations of objects and people. Our mood and state of health and well-being also affect our perceptions. In other words, what we perceive is not a fixed reality, but a subjective experience based upon our own physical, emotional and mental make-up.

The proposition then, that there are energy fields and patterns of which we are – through our five regular senses – unaware, should at least be acceptable to us as a working hypothesis. We still switch on our TV and are happy to use a remote control without ever perceiving anything "coming into" our home or pass from our remote-control device to the TV set! Indeed, we can still use electricity without understanding its nature and governing laws.

Our physical universe is a mixture of both perceivable and imperceivable "gross" matter and more subtle energy fields. Subtle energy fields are the blueprint of physical matter. Our physical body is actually two bodies. The gross physical body, perceivable by the five normal senses, and the subtle – sometimes called etheric – body of which the physical is a precipitation or reflection downwards. The state of the subtle body determines the health of the physical body. In high energy physics terminology, the subtle energy is the "ghost" – energy from which physical matter is derived. Some physicists these days talk of "ghost" electrons, for example. No scientist has ever demonstrated the existence of a "ghost" electron, but theoretically, its existence would seem to be essential to scientific thinking and rationality. In Nature,

★ Pulsor® is a registered trademark of Yao International.

you cannot get "something" for "nothing", for an electron or any sub-atomic particle to exist, there must be something to substantiate it, or give it its energy. That is its "ghost" or subtle counterpart.

According to a theory put forward by Dr. Yao and his research associates, the link point, the window or zero-point between subtle energy and gross physical matter is in the spin and movement of sub-atomic particles.

All sub-atomic particles are in constant motion, they spin and move in three dimensions. One can say that the movement of energy in three dimensions is what makes physical matter "solid" or "real". This physical universe is motion, action, cause and effect – *karma* as the Indian yogi and mystic philosophers call it.

The spin and movement of sub-atomic energy patterns can vary, without any external visible signs of this change in state. In other words, the inner state of kinetic being within sub-atomic matter can vary without the five normal senses being able to perceive any difference. In the high energy physics terms, this duality of our life – light and darkness, heat and cold, happiness and sorrow, life and death – is reflected in the harmony or disharmony of vibration in sub-atomic and allied energy fields which in turn is a reflection of the "polarities" in subtle matter.

In our bodies, the state of our subtle energy determines our degree of health and emotional/mental well-being. In our environment, the harmony or disharmony within subtle energy and the sub-atomic energy patterns, gives rise to the experience of good or bad atmospheres or vibrations.

Our physical bodies then, are comprised of the gross physical of which we are easily aware and the subtle or etheric, the blueprint of the physical, which controls our state of health in the gross physical. Healing can therefore take place in two directions – by controlling the gross physical which will change the polarities in the subtle and/or by changing the polarities in the subtle which will reflect downwards and manifest as the creation of healthy tissues in the gross physical. In practice, those involved in the healing professions, consciously or unconsciously, use a mixture of both.

Subtle Energy Terminology

Throughout the literature on subtle energy topics, we encounter a wide variety of names used in its description. Just as the physical universe displays an endless show of shifting and changing energy patterns, part of which we discern through our senses, so too in the subtle energy fields do we find a spectrum of energies. Different therapies seem to deal with different aspects or areas of these energies. Being beyond our five physical senses, they are more difficult to chart and the names used to describe them can become confusing. We use "subtle energy" to describe all subtle physical and super-physical energies up to the level of mental or thought vibrations. Other terms, some specific, some general are: etheric, Ch'i, prana, bio-energy, auric force field, vortex energy and many more.

Bodily Polarities

All of nature, all our human science, all our activities and those of the cosmos are all underlaid by the principle of duality or polarity. Our universe, our bodies, our emotions, our minds and thoughts are all comprised of gross and subtle energy fields in vibrating and pulsating motion. The cause of this motion is difference – polarity or duality. Even physics tells us that the apparently solid and stationary objects around us are no more than vibrating energy fields of sub-atomic forces – of positive and negative electrical charges, of north and south magnetic fields. Motion exists because of this inequality. Energy, in an eternal cosmic dance, seeks a state of balance. High moves to low, positive runs to negative, clockwise is balanced by anti-clockwise and as it moves, it experiences a force pulling it back to where it was and so it vibrates, orbits or oscillates, like a swing or like the planets.

In Hindu terminology these three states of matter are known as the *Gunas*. *Rajas Guna* is the attribute of activity, of creation, of coming into being. It is springtime, life, restlessness, extrovert, centrifugal, expanding, hot, positive. *Tamas Guna* is the condition of inaction, of destruction, of moving out of being. It is autumn and winter, death, introvert, centipetal, cohering, cold, negative. *Satvas Guna* is the state of balance or harmony between the two. It is peace, equanimity, apparent, changelessness; but it can also be disturbed at any time. Therefore it is temporal and bounded by the transitory nature of existence and is also a state of tension.

The interplay of these three intrinsic forces is manifest in all aspects of existence – inner and outer, in nature as well as our inner lives. The spiritual goal of life lies in transcending the spheres of mind and matter where these three principles hold sway, of moving into the domain of oneness, where peace is intrinsic and not acquired, is absolute – not relative.

But the essence of healing our human ills lies simply in creating harmony amongst the energy patterns of our human constitution. Once this principle is firmly established, then it becomes only a matter of subtle or gross mechanics: of "how?".

As in all energy systems, our human constitution has inherent and specific natural polarities, at both electrical, magnetic and subtle levels. Very briefly, there are three basic subtle energy patterns or circuits in the body, with their in-built, driving polarities. These are:

1. The Mental Circuit. This controls the brain, the head, the main sense organs, the throat and speech. It is particularly strong in intellectual and highly rational people and is linked to these mental faculties; the brain and sense organs being its outward physical manifestation.
2. The Emotional Circuit. This controls the heart, lungs, liver, kidneys, spleen and solar plexus. The energy being derived from that in which feeling and emotion manifest, hence the expressions: "Have a heart" and so on. Emotional upset can result in heart problems or manifest in the solar plexus ("butterflies"). There are numerous connections known to doctors of all callings between our emotional life and their physical manifestation.
3. The Physical Circuit. This controls the pelvic area, including the sex organs, the legs and hands. It is usually the most powerful energy present in physically oriented people.

What Effects These Polarities
Because all energies are interconnected both within ourselves and in our environment, all the processes of life, including just being alive, will effect subtle polarities. These include:
1. Food and Water
2. Air, especially its levels of pollution and ionization.

3. Mental and emotional attitudes and energy, our personality.
4. Electromagnetic radiation
5. Bio-Entrainment
6. The Earth's magnetism and subtle energy fields.

The full effect of these factors cannot easily be discussed in this short chapter and a fuller summary is contained in the book: *Subtle Energy*. Of all these, let us consider in greater detail, the effects of modern, electromagnetic radiation, along with its inevitable counterpart of bio-entrainment.

Vibrational and Electromagnetic Pollution
Polarities in the vortex energy field of the subtle body are also effected by exposure to electromagnetic radiation of all frequencies and wavelengths.

This can be readily understood. Sub-atomic matter is currently seen by modern physics as energy patterns and forces, vibrating at speeds approaching that of light. Indeed, this kinetic energy is an inherent aspect of its being. The forces that hold it all together are also an essential part of its existence. These forces are electromagnetic, gravitational and allied fields. Powerful cosmic rays and particle emissions are already known to alter atomic structure even in a macroscopic sense – molecules and atoms are changed permanently – this is part of the effects of radioactive emissions.

It is highly likely, therefore, that all electromagnetic energy, including light, affects the movement of the energy patterns at sub-atomic levels. Since the sub-atomic energy and electromagnetic energy are of the same nature, they will attract and repel; they will interact; they will not be indifferent to each other.

Sub-atomic and electromagnetic energy are the first physical manifestations of subtle energy. The vibrational states of subtle energy will effect the sub-atomic energy patterns and vice versa. Hence it comes as no surprise to find that electromagnetic energy effects the polarities in our subtle body and causes changes in our level of health and well-being. This need not all be negative, however it does seem that it is only the wavelengths of natural sunlight to which our own bodies and systems are attuned. Outside of these wavelengths, we start having problems.

Modern man is bombarded by electromagnetic radiation of his own creation. One estimate is of 200 millions times more than our ancestors took in from the sun and cosmic sources. Our body and biophysical energies are receivers, conductors and transmitters of this electromagnetic pollution. If you have ever set up a radio aerial you will know how your own body can also behave as an extension to the aerial, simply by your holding the exposed end of the aerial wire.

A powerful demonstration of the body's conductivity and the emission from electrical mains wires can also be made using a TIC-TRACER. The TIC-TRACER bleeps when brought within the induction field surrounding mains cabling and under overhead power lines. If you hold the "insulated" cable in one hand, the body transmits this energy and the bleeping can be detected on the other hand or any other part of the body. The whole body becomes "live".

The electromagnetic energy spectrum can be considered as follows:

10^{29}	10^{26}	10^{18}	10^{16}	1.75×10^{14}	10^{14}	10^{12}	10^{10}–10^4	50–0
						Micro-		
Cosmic	Gamma	X-Rays	Ultra	Visible	Infra	waves	Radio &	ELF
Rays	Rays		Violet	Light	Red	Radar	TV	

the proportions of this diagram being way out and the numbers being the frequencies in (on site) cycles per second (Hertz or Hz).

While studying this list, it is particularly interesting to note that most of the electromagnetic spectrum is already known to be injurious to health. And as we said, if the entire electromagnetic spectrum were represented as a ten thousand mile journey from Cambridge to Peking, the section that humans know of as visible light would measure only six feet.

Other species have senses that detect other parts of this spectrum. Experimenters with American gophers (moles) which dig in beautifully straight lines across lawns and golf courses, throwing up mounds of earths at regular intervals, were able to disorientate them by using an emitter of certain electromagnetic frequencies. The gophers were unable to dig in straight lines and at very high emissions they remained confused and stationary – and died. This would be analogous to putting humans in an environment of strobed and chaotic lighting. It is assumed that gophers are able to sense the lines of force of the earth's natural magnetic and electromagnetic field.

Recent researchers have also found cells with magnetic properties in the foreheads of homing pigeons and ducks, while ELF emissions have been seen to disorientate migrating geese flying overhead. Bees are sensitive to ultra-violet light, while owls can see mice at night through sensitivity to their heat and infra red emanations. Research work at Stanford University has produced evidence of bacteria living symbiotically in the human blood that are magnetically active. Changes in the polarities, caused, for example, by a cut, attract these bacteria to that region of the body, where they are involved in the essential process of forming a clot, to stop bleeding.

An early 1985 article in the New Scientist, describes how the electrical charge on blood cells varies in health and disease. The work of Dr. Harold Saxton Burr on changes in the pure electrical potentials on and around the body's surface show a direct relationship to health, disease and rhythmic body function. Some modern hospital researchers are using electromagnetic and magnetic fields in their treatment of muscular injuries, as well as bone and joint problems, including rheumatism and arthritis, showing once again that the body is sensitive to low level external electrical and electromagnetic activity. In other words the body has electromagnetic energy fields which can be disturbed by environmental electromagnetism.

We are all aware of the harmful effects of certain parts of the electromagnetic spectrum. X-rays, microwave and ultra-violet are particularly well known, other aspects are not so well documented or easy to identify. There is some evidence suggesting that the emanation of microwave ovens, for example, can cause health problems, including cataracts of the eye.

The case of the film set who were irradiated by radioactive fall-out when the wind changed direction during a U.S. Nevada Desert Atomic Explosion Test has become quite well-known. Now, fifteen to twenty years later, many of the cast and film crew are dying or have died of cancer, including John Wayne, Susan Hayward and Clark Gable. Similarly, with the ground zero engineers who were ordered into the area before it was contamination free.

Recent research in the U.K. around the village of Fishpond in Dorset, for example, has related a higher than average incidence of suicide and psychological disturbances amongst people living within the very high electromagnetic induction field surrounding high voltage electricity pylons. In the U.S., a higher than average incidence of leukaemia has been related to high voltage pylons. This field, by the way, can readily be detected with a TIC-TRACER up to one or two hundred feet away. Standing under these pylons personally makes me feel "creepy" and nauseous.

There are many such cases that can be quoted. The point is that this kind of electromagnetic pollution may not show up in serious illness for as long as fifteen to twenty years after the event. Furthermore, it is very difficult to quantify the effect of continual bombardment by low intensity electromagnetic radiation such as TV and radio broadcasting and ordinary mains circuit emissions in domestic and commercial properties.

There have recently been a number of reports indicating a statistically significant proportion of miscarriages and embryonic deformities amongst expectant mothers working on VDU's – computers and word processors etc. Embryo deformities can be the result of chromosomal damage. Chromosomal damage can be caused by electromagnetic radiation. VDU's (and TV's) emit electromagnetic radiation. Chromosomal damage becomes most rapidly apparent in cells which are dividing rapidly. Embryonic cells are naturally dividing rapidly – this is what constitutes their growth and the more subtle organizational, information-encoded, subtle blueprints are naturally operating at high 'capacity' during embryological development. Therefore, small doses of radiation will have greater damaging effect on embryos over a short period of time, than on adults. Moreover, the total structure of the organism is derived from the chromosomes, so any embryonic, chromosomal damage will also be liable to cause deformities. And finally, one cause of miscarriage is deformity – the body's natural mechanisms detect problems and the foetus is aborted. The effect of VDU's on expectant mothers is therefore quite readily understandable.

There are many parallels, too, in other areas of environmental pollution. DDT, for example, was heralded as a boon to pest control. However, it was later found to be harmful to human health and the recommended quantities to be used by farmers were drastically reduced. Later on, as it became evident that DDT is both stored in the body over long periods, is both poisonous and carcinogenic, and is also non-biodegradable so that it remains in the soil year after year – it became a 'non-recommended' (not illegal) chemical.

Similarly, what is discounted today as unharmful electromagnetic radiation may, in the light of further evidence, prove to have highly injurious effects on our long-term health and well-being. It would be interesting to have accurate statistics on the relationship between the high incidence of cancer and heart disease and the build up in usage over the last three decades of electrical appliances, computer, VDU and electronic equipment and especially TV and radio signal broadcasting and receiving. Workers in the field of energy balancing can relate reversals and disturbances in these subtle centres to electromagnetic bombardment. This is evidence enough for them, though it may not satisfy the more conventional and conservative mind.

It is not just the emissions of electrical appliances and TV/radio broadcasting, however, that cause problems. All metal objects act as aerials for electromagnetic radiation, just like the TV aerial on the roof of one's home. Electrical currents are induced in tooth-fillings, buckles, jewellery and zippers on our body as well as in all the metal work in our homes and offices – electrical wiring, water pipes and, most importantly, in the coiled springs inside mattresses. Since we spend one third of our life asleep, this factor is of some importance.

Bio-Entrainment

The bio-energy, subtle force field or aura of the body is also effected by sympathetic resonance with similar force fields. This partly explains, for example, why husband and wife who have lived together for many years can take on very similar features in both physical appearance, as well as in mental and emotional attitudes. They are living within each other's aura and their vibrations become attuned to each other.

We are also affected by the presence of other people on a day to day basis. Note also how moods can take over an entire crowd or room full of people. We talk, too, of atmospheres – good or bad – that build up amongst groups of people. We also find that certain places, homes or individual rooms have 'good' or 'bad' vibrations and affect us accordingly.

When this effect is long term, it creates a habit in our body, known as 'bio-entrainment', a form of subtle energy resonance, and while we may be happy to be uplifted by good vibrations, we would prefer to avoid the drag of the negative.

The experience of the majority of Pulsor users is that they amplify the body's natural aura, providing a strong, protective force field in which one is more able to influence others than have them influence us. When in places with a negative atmosphere, users report feeling cocooned and cushioned against its potential effect on them.

Entrainment of brain and body functions can also occur from electromagnetic radiation. The heart, brain and muscles all emit signals from less than one cycle per second to over a hundred thousand cycles per second. These signals form the basis of electrocardiograms and electroencephalograms. Amidst all this electrical activity, four predominant brain wave patterns can be identified:

Delta	0.5 to 3Hz	Deep sleep, higher states of consciousness
Theta	4 to 7Hz	Reverie, dream states
Alpha	8 to 13Hz	Passive, blank, relaxed, meditation
Beta	14 to 30Hz	Thinking, active mind and/or body

ELF (extremely low frequency) electromagnetic emissions at these frequencies are thus likely to be psycho-active. That is, they can affect your mood. It is said that the USSR and the USA have both developed and use such weapons. They call it 'world mood manipulation' and 'psychotronic warfare'.

A recent TV documentary revealed that the Soviet Union has built the three largest broadcasting stations ever designed. From these stations are broadcast a pulsed electromagnetic signal that is receivable as a click on a shortwave radio. This is the most powerful electromagnetic signal ever broadcast. The given code name is 'Woodpecker' and both the U.S.A. and Europe – but not the U.S.S.R. – are targets for this emission. The U.S.A. have responded by building a similar transmitter, the signals from which are bounced off the ionosphere, but the Soviet Union now have many years research behind them on psycho-active, electromagnetic frequencies.

Very little research has really been made in the West, but in Russia and Eastern Europe, hundreds of experiments have shown that electromagnetic fields may cause a host of health problems, including blood disorders, hypertension, heart attacks, headaches, sexual disfunction, drowsiness and nervous exhaustion. The book: *Electromagnetic Fields and Life* by A.S. Presman from the Department of Biophysics, Moscow University, describes in detail many such experiments. It was first published in Russian in 1968 and translated into English in 1970.

As a result of their experimentation, the Soviet Union have strict rules over the amount and duration of emission from radio transmitters and radars that a person can safely absorb. The West has only an informal, non-legal guideline set in 1966 by the U.S. American Standards Institute. The Soviet criterion is one thousand times tougher than this for workers and ten thousand times more for civilians. Clearly, the Russians believe that even small doses of electromagnetic smog, over time, can do great harm.

In 1962, the CIA discovered that the Soviets were beaming microwaves into the U.S. embassy in Moscow, deliberately aimed at the U.S. ambassador's office from two buildings across the street. It was .002 of the intensity that the American guideline called dangerous The CIA set up experiments to duplicate the irradiation on monkeys and within three weeks there were adverse effects on the animals' nervous and immune systems. Embassy officials, however were not informed of the irradiation. Instead they were asked to give blood samples to 'test for a disease in Moscow's water'. These tests revealed that about a third had a white blood cell count almost fifty percent higher than normal – often a symptom of severe infection and also a characteristic of leukaemia.

In 1976, the U.S. State Department declared the Moscow embassy an 'unhealthful post', and metal window screens were put up to shield against the microwave beams. But this was fourteen years after their discovery. Today, those former embassy personnel exhibit a higher rate of cancer than the American average, and two U.S. embassadors in Moscow subjected to this radiation have died of cancer.

We relate these incidents concerning the 'superpowers', not in any political spirit or wish to create divisions amongst our fellow humans, but simply because they highlight certain problem areas. Some of these incidents sound almost unbelievable, yet so does the creation of nuclear devices designed to destroy life completely for the sake of political or economic ideals. Why do humans inflict such suffering on themselves?

Similarly, it seems likely that part of the computer and video 'junkie' syndrome, affecting many people, has its roots in an addiction to the electromagnetic radiations and voltage potentials around the VDU. And finally let us add that subtle energy polarities are reversed by crossing the earth magnetic lines of force, this being one of the causes of jet-lag and premature ageing in air-line pilots and air-hostesses. It is one of the reasons why an east-west or west-east flight has a worse effect than a north-south journey.

DOWSING & THE DETECTION OF SUBTLE ENERGIES

By their very nature, subtle energies cannot easily, if at all, be brought under the microscope or into the laboratory for scrutiny. In fact, the subtle energies of one's own being must be experienced in order to appreciate them. Some psychically gifted people are able to directly perceive these energies up to a certain level, depending upon the individual. This, for example, is how such therapies as acupuncture and polarity therapy must have had their origins. But for most of us, the technique used to tap our unconscious knowledge of these energies is known as dowsing.

This is a wide ranging subject, but basically, our unconscious and superconscious mind know the 'answers' (relatively speaking) to all our questions and problems. Dowsing is a technique by which we explicitly or implicitly ask our unconscious mind a 'question' and receive the 'reply' by way of water-divining rods, by means of a pendulum, by radionic machines, through such systems as kinesiology or muscle testing and in other similar ways.

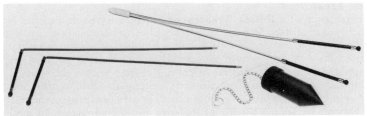

Acu-Pulsor Pendulum and Swivel-Handled & V-Shaped Dowsing Rods

We recommend that you read up on this fascinating subject (there is chapter on it in *Subtle Energy*), because there are many aspects to it, but for assessing the condition of bodily and environmental energies, we personally use the Acu-Pulsor Pendulum because of its constant polarity, and for dowsing rods, we use two highly sensitive pairs, carefully hand-made in plastic-coated steel. With these, you can measure the extent of auras, discover underground water or minerals, map the flow of ley lines or earth energies and so on. A large majority of people can learn to dowse with reasonable accuracy and consistency, because these energies are a part of the constitution of all of us, and it is certainly worth a try. It will develop your intuitive awareness, too.

★*WHAT ARE PULSORS?*

Pulsors are a unique blend of modern physics with ancient healing wisdom. They have an activity in the interface between subtle energies and the sub-atomic and are literally able to change and amplify the vibrations and auras of people and places! **Pulsors** are at the leading edge of Aquarian science. They are truely the forerunners of twenty-first century technology.

Dr George Yao, now a Naturopathic Doctor, but previously an aerospace engineer, created the first **Pulsors** fifteen years ago during his work with Acupuncture, Polarity Therapy and Bio-Energy Field balancing.

A **Pulsor** is a solid-state, composite of micro-crystals, arranged in specific patterns, giving it the ability to resonate with and harmonize subtle energy vibrations, thereby amplifying the personal aura, protecting from environmental influences and creating a warm and nourishing atmosphere in which to live.

★ Pulsor® is a registered trademark of Yao International.

They are bio-energy, receiver/transmitters with ultra-wide wavebands. Just as quartz crystals are used in electronics for their fixed frequency resonance, so too can other crystals be used for their activity through the curtain – beyond the sub-atomic particles – into more subtle energy.

In people – this activity manifests as healing, as an increased feeling of well-being and as a warm, protective umbrella against external influences, including polarity reversals caused by the continuous, low-energy bombardment of electromagnetic radiation from electrical cabling and appliances, as well as radio and TV broadcasting. **In places and homes** – a positive, nourishing atmosphere can be created, over-riding any previous negative vibrations and amplifying the positive. Relationships become more harmonious, businesses and healing practices prosper, energy flows more freely and lovingly – and everyone feels better.

Pulsor Treatment

The experience of a **Pulsor Treatment** can be very profound and is almost invariably one of deep and uplifting relaxation, where healing continues long after the therapy session. We have had a number of people who can see the enhanced flow of energy within themselves as coloured patterns, especially through and around the chakras or energy centres within the spine.

Acupuncturists, radionic practitioners, osteopaths and anyone doing body work or any form of natural healing, can all benefit and protect themselves and their patients by adding the use of **Pulsors** into their practice. In the home or office, **Pulsors** can improve the quality of life and being.

Those working in close proximity to electronic equipment, telephone switchboards, VDU's, computers etc., need **Pulsor** protection to avoid polarity reversals. Those who have worked in such environments for many years often experience profound relief after **Pulsor** treatment and feel better than they have felt for a long time.

Who Should Use Them?

Well..... everybody! The polarity reversal effects of electro-magnetic pollution cannot be overstressed. It adds an insidious, dirtiness into one's environment reflecting as disharmony and general malaise in all aspects of life. If used with understanding, **Pulsors** can help bring back the sparkle to life. Other factors that can cause polarity reversals are: food, water, air, other people(!), places ... almost anything! **Pulsors**, therefore, are our protective umbrella.

Applications

1. **Wearing personally for aura nourishment and amplification**, stress relief, energy balancing, and protection from environmental electro-magnetic pollution and the ambient atmospheres of places and people. This is particularly helpful to medical and healing practitioners of any kind who feel drained of energy after a day of seeing patients. Also, to help remedy specific ailments – pains, sore throats, stomach pains, cramps or more serious problems.

2. **On the electricity, water and gas input points** to your house to make their effect positive or harmless.

3. **On the telephone**, to alleviate the energy drain caused by its use. Also, **TV's and refridgerators** etc.

4. **For relaxation and therapy** – either professionally, within a family and friends, or self-applied.

5. **To remove the negative effect of electrical charge** lodged in metal jewellery, tooth fillings, belt buckles, zippers, etc, that gets there from contact with light switches, electrical appliances and electrical currents induced by radio and TV broadcasting.

6. **Around your bed.** The coiled springs of most mattresses act as superb amplifying aerials for TV and radio broadcast signals which upset our polarities whilst we sleep. **Pulsors** provide a warm nourishing and protective sleeping environment.

7. **Around your home and office,** to provide a good atmosphere in which to live and work harmoniously.

8. **For international travellers** including air-hostesses and pilots. Jet lag is partly due to the continuous polarity reversals caused by crossing the earth's magnetic grid. **Pulsors** provide the necessary protection and jet lag is alleviated. This also explains why crossing east-west or west-east is worse in effect than a journey north-south or south-north.

Choosing Which Pulsor(s)
Pulsors have three frequencies, coloured for convenience.

Blue Pulsors resonate with our mental energies.
Green Pulsors resonate with emotional energies.
Red Pulsors resonate with the physical body.

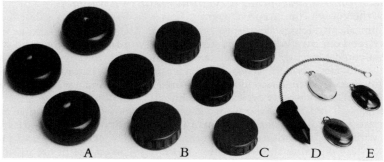

Torroid Pulsors (A), 2" diameter; Professional Pulsors (B), 1¾" diameter; Compact Professional Pulsors (C), 1½" diameter; Acu-Pulsor Pendulum & Acupoint Stimulator (D); Pulsor Pendants (E).

There are a number of different types of Pulsor for different applications, including **Pendants** for personal protection that contain all the frequencies.

CHAPTER SIX

NATURAL FERTILITY AWARENESS INTO THE 21st CENTURY

Man and Nature

Nature has a way of keeping its own balance, of solving its own problems. And Man is not separate from Nature, he is a part of its rhythm, caught up in its dynamic interplay. Man may think that he can control Nature, but this would seem to be a very narrow viewpoint. No person knows for sure what will happen to him within the next five minutes, or, indeed, what even his thoughts will be. We are all inherently bound up in the great cosmic Mystery, our 'freedom' thus being greatly limited.

Man's creation of environmental problems and his attempts to solve them may therefore be seen as an evolution of his understanding, a necessary step in his movement towards a technology that is in harmony and not antagonism with Nature. As man's awareness, consciousness and even love (spiritual) evolve, his selfishness decreases and he moves into a more harmonious understanding of his position in the cosmos. At the same time, through negative feedback, Nature compels him to clean up his own dirty messes.

There are many examples of this process – the population of the human race being but one. Through an increased understanding of health and disease, the population of our earth is increasing dramatically. This factor, along with the normal social reasons for wishing to avoid a pregnancy have led to our development of an array of devices to prevent conception. Nor is it necessary in modern times to produce a large family on the assumption that some will die in childhood or early adulthood. These days, most of us consider it unlucky for someone not to live at least past fifty; while to live up to sixty, seventy or eighty is considered nothing unusual.

Population, Contraception & Natural Fertility Awareness

All of the known contraceptive devices, however, have negative side-effects – anatomical, physiological and/or psychological. How good it would be if we understood our own body signals so well that a woman knew when and when not she could conceive? This understanding is not so far from us as many would believe. In fact, modern research has identified many natural indicators of fertility that can be understood and monitored by any woman wishing to know more about her own body cycles. The techniques are known as Natural Fertility Awareness – and it is a knowledge desperately needed by the human race. Scientists have come to understand many of these indicators so well, that when used with care, conception can be prevented at a level of 99% – comparable with that of the Pill – with the 1% relating more to incorrect use of the methods, rather than its fallibility.

Natural Fertility Awareness (NFA) – also called Natural Family Planning (NFP) and Natural Birth Control – is a thousand miles removed from the highly unsafe 'rhythm method'. It is based on an interpretation of natural signs of ovulation – the very short time in a cycle when conception can occur. These signs, *which are directly linked to the hormonal system – the same system which makes the Pill such a safe method of contraception* – include: a rise in the basal body temperature, the condition and volume of cervical mucus, the presence of certain hormones (especially LH – Luteinizing Hormone) in the urine, the condition of the cervix, and other more minor indicators. It is modern, scientific and totally in keeping with the move away from drugs in the minds and practice of a increasing number of people. Many doctors, even, are not yet aware of its potential – often confusing it with the rhythm method. We believe that it should be taught in schools – knowledge of such vitally important changes in a woman's body should be made easily available.

NFA is *about* people and *for* people. We all have a body – and we all have a right to a knowledge of that body and to an awareness of its functioning. This kind of knowledge is not the province of medical people alone. This means that anyone interested can learn to understand or teach NFA – a nursing or medical background is not required.

A Great Help For Couples Having a Problem Conceiving

With statistics of one in six couples having difficulty in conception, any system that increases their chances without resorting to drugs is to be welcomed with open arms. Natural Fertility Awareness methods are unique in that they can also help to achieve as well as avoid pregnancy. It seems quite probable, therefore, that they will become the major means of family planning used in the 21st century, especially when the available fertility indicators include new hormonal urine tests and are augmented by other domestic products of modern technology, such as *OVIA* – a new product from the Wholistic Research Company of Cambridge.

The Hormone Sequence

The menstrual cycle is precisely controlled by hormones secreted by the ovaries and the pituitary gland. In simplistic terms, and starting our description just after menstruation, the pituitary gland, (the master gland in the brain that controls the other endocrine glands), produces Follicle Stimulating Hormone (FSH). FSH stimulates just one follicle (a sort of cellular envelope) in the ovary to produce an ovum, the female egg. As the follicle develops, it produces the hormone oestrogen. As the level of oestrogen rises, it stimulates the pituitary to secrete a surge of the Luteinizing Hormone (LH). LH further stimulates the active follicle and within 4 to 64 hours, it breaks open to release the ovum. The ovum now has about 12 to 24 hours of life in which it can be fertilized.

The level of oestrogen now drops off and the remaining follicle produces the hormone progesterone and, if conception does not occur, the level of progesterone drops off until the uterine lining is shed at menstruation, the cycle starting all over again.

Ovulation can thus occur only once during the cycle, due to hormone levels. Fraternal twins can occur if both ovaries produce an ovum, but since the LH surge occurs only once in a cycle, the second ovulation can only happen a few hours after the first. Identical twins occur when the ovum divides into two after fertilization, thus producing embryos with identical genetic material.

The hormone contraceptive Pill contains both oestrogen and progesterone, which, when taken on a daily basis, maintains a non-ovulatory, non-menstrual condition.

Infertile and Fertile Phases
There are thus four distinct phases within the menstrual cycle.

1. The period of menstruation, which is usually infertile, but not always so, especially in those with short cycles.

2. The pre-ovulatory infertile phase, before ovulation occurs.

3. The fertile phase, around ovulation.

4. The post-ovulatory infertile phase, after which menstruation occurs and the cycle restarts.

Reports of pregnancy occuring due to making love during menstruation are due either to very short cycles when ovulation occurs soon after the end of the period or most probably to blood spotting that can occur at the time of ovulation, so that the supposed menstruation was not menstruation at all but a time of maximum fertility.

Bearing in mind that sperm can live up to a maximum of five days within the vagina and uterus and that the ovum has a life of up to 24 hours, it is therefore possible to assess quite accurately when a woman is likely or unlikely to conceive.

NATURAL FERTILITY INDICATORS
What then are these external indicators, that accompany the changes in hormone levels, and let us know when ovulation is occuring?

Natural Fertility Indicators – 1. Cervical Mucus: Type & Quantity
Just after menstruation the vagina is normally dry. Any mucus is dry, even flaky, and the opening to the uterus is plugged by dryish mucus. The condition in the vagina is also acid and hostile to sperm life. As the oestrogen level rises, prior to ovulation, the mucus becomes greater in quantity as well as being wetter and stretchy – like the white of a raw egg. It also becomes alkaline and friendly towards towards sperm. This wetness reaches a peak just before the LH surge, which stimulates ovulation. After ovulation, the mucus again becomes thicker and dry once again. Hence, by observing the condition of the mucus and bearing in mind the relative lifetimes of sperm and ovum, an assessment of fertility can be made.

Natural Fertility Indicators – 2. Cervical State
Following the pattern of the cervical mucus, there are also associated changes in the cervix itself, the cervix being the lower part of the uterus (the womb) including the opening into the vagina. The cervix becomes softer, higher up in the abdomen and its aperture opens to allow the passage of sperm, swimming up the wet coating of slippery, fertile-type mucus.

Natural Fertility Indicators – 3. Basal Body Temperature
The rise in the level of progesterone immediately after ovulation causes a marked rise in the basal body temperature of about .1–.2°C or .2–.4°F. This is

maintained until menstruation and a fall-off in the level of progesterone. The post-ovulatory infertile phase can thus be readily noted. The temperature is taken first thing in the morning, before getting out of bed, with a special fertility thermometer – a highly accurate, easily readable, clinical thermometer with divisions of .1 or less.

Natural Fertility Indicators – 4. Luteinizing Hormone Test
The presence of LH in the urine coincides with the LH surge that stimulates ovulation. Thus, by using a simple, domestic dip-stick test that goes blue when positive, the LH surge can readily be detected. This, especially when combined with the rise in basal body temperature, gives a very accurate indication of the post-ovulatory infertile phase. More importantly, it also indicates the fertile time as it is occurring – a real help to those having trouble conceiving.

Natural Fertility Indicators – 5. Other Signs
Blood spotting and/or a sharp pain in the region of the ovaries (mittelschmerz) around the time of ovulation, tenderness and swelling of the breasts, plus subjective feelings and intuition are also minor indicators of ovulation. Women who are in tune with themselves often come to know intuitively when they are fertile. Their partner, too, may be aware of a stronger attraction at this time.

By correlating all these signs, therefore, on a chart or the small electronic device known as OVIA, (a friend of ours recently christened it the 'Love Computer'), an accurate assessment can be made of the likelihood of conception occuring should you make love at that time.

A Positive Step Towards Knowledge of One's Body
At first sight, the monitoring of these natural indicators might seem to be a hassle. However, after a learning period, it becomes no more of a problem than remembering to brush one's teeth or take account of the weather when choosing which clothes to wear. Furthermore, the intimate knowledge and understanding of one's own body rhythms more than outweighs any minor initial inconvenience while learning. Finally, many couples have reported that the shared knowledge of the cycle and the required, loving co-operation generated, have added new dimensions and understanding to their relationship. Natural Family Planning is also cheaper than other methods.

Learning how to interpret the various signs can be done from a book only if you easily absorb information in that way. Even so, interpretation of oddities in the signs may need the help of someone experienced. Here, OVIA is a useful device, since it is intelligent enough to assess, automatically, the common and not-so-common oddities. The number of NFP teachers is also growing, but there is still room for many more. And if you learn from a friend, make sure they know what they are talking about!

Stress and Ovulation
Many women have noticed that stress can cause extremely long cycles or even the absence of menstruation altogether. The reason again has a hormonal aspect. Another endocrine gland, the hypothalamus, also in the brain, acts as the body's environment monitor. It is secretions from the hypothalamus, for example, that

cause you to sweat when you get hot, in order to cool you down. Similarly, under stress, the production of FSH is inhibited by a secretion from the hypothalamus and hence the cycle is extended or never reaches an oestrogen peak.

Reliability & Statistical Studies

The rules for assessing the levels of fertility throughout a cycle have been thoroughly tested over the last twenty years. Probably the most significant of these was the internationally conducted Fairfield trial in 1977, which showed quite conclusively that the effectiveness of the combined indicator methods was greater than 99% when used correctly. This figure is corroborated by studies conducted both before and since.

Natural Fertility Awareness Education Centre: Tuition and Correspondence Course

All the statistical studies concerning the reliability of natural methods of birth control have also shown that the failure rate increases in direct relation to the **quality of both practice and teaching**. Although *OVIA* should improve this situation by taking much of the responsibility of assessment onto its own self, we wholeheartedly agree that to really absorb this knowledge, it is better to be professionally taught, rather than attempting to teach oneself from a book. In the context of a lifetime and considering what is at stake, it is indeed only a small investment of time and resources.

It is for this reason, therefore, that we have introduced a **Natural Fertility Awareness Correspondence Course** for both users and prospective teachers, and have started an international Natural Fertility Awareness Education Centre. At the present time of writing (January 1986), it is only small, but the interest we are receiving is tremendous, for obvious reasons, and we envisage considerable expansion of our facilities in the years ahead.

So this short chapter should be taken only as a lead in to the subject, not in any way as a tutor. Many people, for example, hearing that there is a temperature rise around the time of ovulation begin taking their temperature. Not knowing how to do it correctly or interpret their findings, they can often make no sense of their recordings and become discouraged. This is especially the case with couples who are having problems conceiving and are given misleading or incomplete information by their doctor.

Further Information and Useful Products

There are a number of books available on Fertility Awareness and Natural Family Planning. In our own book: *Natural Fertility Awareness* we have tried to be clear, simple and complete in our description of the methods and there are other good books too, of course.

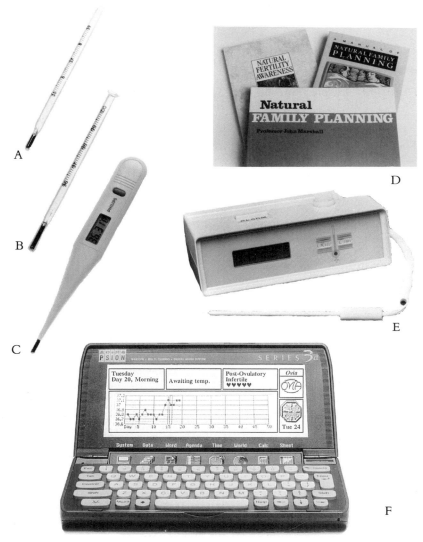

Other useful products also available include **FERTILITY THERMO-METERS** (A & B) with an extended accuracy, including a rather neat **DIGITAL CLINICAL THERMOMETER** from Becton Dickinson (C), a range of books and charts on Natural Fertility Awareness, infertility, birth control and allied topics (D); the **RITE-TIME** (E), which detects the temperature shift and the post-ovulatory infertile phase; and finally the latest version of *OVIA* (F), which ties everything together in a small hand-held, very user-friendly, personal organizer, helping you achieve or avoid conception according to your needs.

CHAPTER SEVEN

BOUNCERS – AEROBIC REBOUNDING

How This Simple Exercise Can Stimulate Your Metabolism, Keeping You Fit, Healthy And Feeling Good
The Most Efficient Form of Exercise Yet Devised by Man

There are innumerable systems for keeping fit, but according to modern research, there is one form of exercise that is more complete than any other. It is called aerobic rebounding and it consists of simple, ordinary exercises performed on a firm mini–trampoline – a bouncer or rebounder. And there are scientific reasons, too, why such exercise is so good for you.

What is Exercise and What is a Good Exercise?
Exercise is a process by which the cells of the body are placed under a controlled stress. They are thus stimulated to reach a higher degree of metabolic efficiency as well as to increase in vigour, strength and vitality. Our physical body consists of these cells, and interconnecting structures, along with fluids, nerve impulses and more subtle energies, and the stronger and more vital the individual cells become, the better we feel and the fitter we are, one of the secrets of good health lies in building healthy body tissues or cell structures in all parts of our body.

Most forms of exercise are good at stimulating particular body tissues, but leave aside the strengthening of others. An efficient form of exercise therefore will be one which reaches every cell in the body.

If you analyze the mechanisms of jogging, swimming, tennis, weight-lifting and most gym-training you will find that the cellular stimulation is created in certain parts of the body only, by working particular muscles of the body against gravity or against another resistive force. At no time during the exercise cycle are *all* the cells of the body *simultaneously* stimulated. Such exercise is therefore only partial, for however long you may continue it. For this reason, keep fit programmes contain a number of different forms of exercise in order to strengthen and vitalize as many parts of the body as possible.

Rebounding Exercises Every Body Cell
When exercise is performed on a sprung-mat, however, the situation becomes very different because you are now combining the force of gravity with those of acceleration and deceleration. To the body, however, *these forces combine, appearing as just one rhythmically changing force, exerted simultaneously in every cell of the body*. When you are at the top of a bounce the body cells are under a zero gravity stress, when at the bottom of a bounce, the rapid deceleration combines with the force of gravity to create a stimulation to the body tissues of up to twice the force of gravity. It is for this reason that even the North American Space Agency (NASA) have researched the power of simple bouncing exercises, declaring them to be *the most efficient form of exercise yet devised by man*.

This rhythmic, simultaneous, stimulation of every body cell has been shown by physiologists and trainers to provide some remarkable effects.

Body cells, although of many different kinds, all possess the same basic properties. Each requires oxygen and nutrients for its continued well-being. They have a most remarkable membrane which maintains an electrical differential as well as a potassium, magnesium and phosphate/ sodium and chloride differential across its surface. Each cell, too, has an intelligence. It contains within itself, through its complex nucleus, a blueprint for re-building the entire body, though it only draws from that intelligence what it needs for its own local functioning.

Rebounding Increases Muscular Strength

When cells are stressed or exercised below the point of rupture, they become strong, well toned; when they have little work to perform, their condition degenerates and they atrophy. The body's strength results from the combined overall strength of trillions of cells. Rebound exercise thus creates muscular, tissue and organ strength through the stressing effect of each cell created by the changing of gravitational, accelerating and decelerating forces, rather than by the work-oriented aspects of other form of exercise. It is sometimes a point not immediately grasped that even muscular strength can be developed not only by work or by using the muscle, but also by the gentle stressing of gravitational rebounding.

This factor has an additional advantage, too, in that work-orientated, stress-stimulation exercises such as jogging, swimming etc., can over-stress areas of the body, resulting in structural injuries because of the *sudden* occurrence of stress. Consider for example, the back, tendon and knee problems of runners and joggers who continually land on a hard, unyielding surface. With bouncing, the cells are stimulated without the sudden stress that can result in injury. It is for similar reasons, too, that bouncing is used in remedial exercise after accidents and injuries, to help promote strength and healing. Even just sitting on a bouncer and rhythmically moving up and down is of help in cases where more strenuous movement is impossible or ill-advised.

Bouncers are thus found to be of great assistance for exercising older people or in re-building strength after injuries or operations. They are frequently recommended by physiotherapists and are used extensively in rehabilitation centres.

Rebounding Stimulates Lymphatic Elimination of Cellular Toxins and Waste Materials

Our body cells are in a continual state of renewal. Some cells last only twenty-four hours, like our red blood cells. Others last longer, even many years. Our brain cells do not renew themselves – we simply have innumerable spare ones to replace those that die. It is thought, however, that running out of spare cells is one of the causes of senility and the slowness and loss of memory often associated with old age. Modern research, however, does point out that although dead brain cells cannot be brought back to function, the remaining cells can be stimulated to grow new interconnections.

It is as necessary for the body to be able to get rid of the broken down products and toxins of old cells, as it is for nutrients to reach the tissues for the creation of new ones. In addition, normal healthy cells will require nutrition, whilst also needing their excretory, waste products to be taken away. This is essential for health and well-being. This transport of toxins away from the cells, into the blood stream and out through the kidneys, skin and lungs is accomplished initially through the *lymph* system. Lymph and its associated lymphocytes (cells) is the fluid which bathes all the body cells. It is a loosely structured system that extends throughout the body, but does contain tubules and valves similar to the circulatory system.

Rhythmic bouncing helps to move these toxins out of the cells into the lymph fluid, and thence into the blood stream, on their way to excretion and elimination from the body. The presence of unreleased toxins leads to cellular degeneration, disease and deposits. The flap-like valves within the lymphatic tubules are stimulated and strengthened and vitality is restored.

Rebounding as an Aerobic-Plus Exercise

The aerobic nature of rebounding should also be considered. Cells need oxygen to burn carbohydrates, fats and proteins for the release of nutrients and energy. This process requires the absorption of atmospheric oxygen and results in the release of carbon dioxide, the gaseous exchange taking place, of course, in the lungs. Any exercise, therefore, which increases the flow of oxygen to the cells is rightly considered aerobic. Note, however, that the problem of getting oxygen to the cells is not one of *supply* to the body – the atmosphere is normally full of it – it is one of *delivery* to the cells. That is, a strong cardio-vascular system is required. Exercise designed only to stimulate cardio-vascular efficiency, however, is not going to be as effective as an all round exercise which stimulates the cells themselves to be able to *absorb* both the oxygen and the nutrients. Bouncing, of course, does just this, something which other, even more energetic forms of aerobic exercising, may not be able to accomplish.

Rebounding Is Fun

Exercise is an activity most of us feel we should do more of, but often lack the will-power or enthusiasm. To all except 'fitness-freaks', exercise can be inordinately boring, resulting in our giving it up after only a short period of time. James R. White, a rehabilitation researcher at the University of California at San Diego, conducted an interesting study of the different kinds of domestic exercise. Apart from the increase of fitness and decrease in weight of most of his subjects, the drop-out rate in a long-term follow up study revealed that while only 5% of the cyclists and 31% of the runners were still exercising, 58% of the bouncers were still bouncing.

The answer given was simple. Bouncing was both easy and fun. You don't need any special clothes and you don't even need to go outside. In the privacy of your own home, you can exercise in any clothes you like. You can watch TV or listen to music. Bouncing is definitely an exercise-saving exercise. And kids just love it, they are kept amused for hours.

Rebounding Increases Skeletal Strength, Improves Eyesight, Enhances Learning Ability

The effect of cellular stimulation can have many other effects, also documented by researchers. Skeletal strength is increased – bone is also comprised of very special cells – and the demineralization due to age is retarded or stopped. This stimulating effect of gravity on the calcium content of bones was first observed when astronauts returned from the zero gravity conditions of only fourteen days in space with a 15% loss in bone-mass.

Eyesight has also been reported as improved, due to the strengthening of the ocular muscles and tissues of the eye. In fact, after only a few minutes of bouncing one's vision often seems clearer. Colours are seen more vibrantly and you feel better.

Educationalists too, have reported marked improvement in the learning ablity and emotional stability of children who bounce regularly. It seems that every aspect of health can be improved by the gentle or vigorous stimulation of rebounding.

Deciding on a Suitable Bouncer

When purchasing a bouncer, you need to watch out for a number of factors: a cheap bouncer can let you down rather badly! Firstly, the frame must be continuous with leg supports firmly welded in position. The legs should have rubber ferrels on the end to save making holes in your lawn or carpet and should be tightly secured into place. The mat should be evenly sprung and not too loose. The springs must be fixed *securely* into the mat. With some inexpensive bouncers, the edges of the springs wear holes in the mats and they fall apart quite rapidly. The springs should also be arranged in V-orientations. A parallel arrangement is unsuitable because it does not provide the sense of being drawn into the centre, leaving you with a feeling of insecurity. And finally, the cover should be of a suitable material, padded on the inside to avoid friction against the springs wearing holes in it.

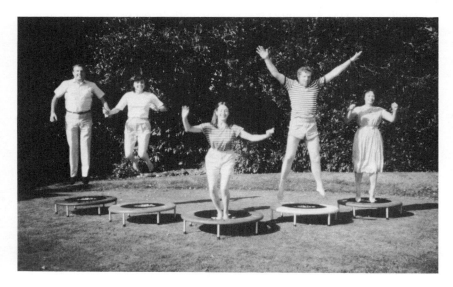

The PT Bouncer which is stocked by the Wholistic Research Company has all these features and is available in a 40″ diameter. Smaller bouncers are somewhat less bouncier!

47

CHAPTER EIGHT

TIP-U-UP's

On The Benefits Of Having Your Feet Higher Than Your Head.
A Strong Healthy Back is One of the Keys to Good Health

On The Effect of Gravity and the Use of TIP-U-UP's

From the moment you enter this world, until the moment you leave it, the pull of gravity is one of the most dominating and influential forces in your physical life on earth.

Most of the results of gravity's stress on the human body are obvious .... baggy eyes, drooping jowls, strained necks, round shoulders, sunken chests, dropping busts, bad backs, prolapse organs, sagging abdomens, hanging buttocks, varicose veins, swollen ankles and fallen arches!

In addition, if you stand and sit all day, and then sleep with your head on top of a pillow at night, gravity hinders the flow of blood upward to your head .... where poor circulation threatens the well being of your eyes-vision, ears-hearing, gums-teeth, brain-memory, scalp-hair and skin-complexion.

Lying down with your feet higher than your head and heart is a recognized scientific means of using the law of gravity to benefit your youth and vitality. Utilizing gravity to uplift your body, instead of pulling it down, is an ancient health and beauty technique, and has long been an integral part of Hatha Yoga disciplines. TIP-U-UP's are modern aids that now make this practice an enjoyable experience for you. TIP-U-UP's are the most practical way of lying down with your head lower than your heart.

Lying on a TIP-U-UP reverses gravity's pull on your entire body. It is a natural position for revitalizing your legs and feet, relaxing your neck, stretching your spine, calming your mind and rejuvenating your body.

So – put your feet up – but don't try having a cup of tea simultaneously!

THE CUSHION TIP-U-UP

This unique idea in super-firm foam gives you a four-in-one, highly useful *and* healthy piece of inexpensive furniture.

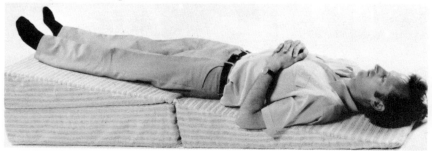

★ **The Cushion TIP-U-UP** was created for fitness, furniture and fun, for your body and mind, for your family and friends, for your home and office.

★ As a TIP-U-UP, it tips you up by 14″ at the foot.
★ At 72″ × 22″ × 7″, it provides you with an extra bed.
★ At 36″ × 22″ × 14″, it makes an ottoman.
★ At a folded right angle against the wall, it makes a lounge seat.

The **Cushion TIP-U-UP** is only available as the raw foam pieces themselves, for you to cover or not, as you feel inclined.

THE GENTLE TIP-U-UP

Standing 18″ at the foot, the portable, **Gentle TIP-U-UP** is designed to fold up and go behind your sofa or in a cupboard. The 18mm thick, birch multi-ply board, padded and covered in an easily cleaned brown vinyl fabric, folds to half its 75″ × 16″ size, while the mild steel frame comes apart by undoing the wing nuts. The foot end also has a strap to allow use as a home exerciser. The **Gentle TIP-U-UP** is similar, but not identical to the Slanting Board discussed by Dr. Jensen in his books. A sheet of ten exercises suggested by Dr. Jensen, is provided.

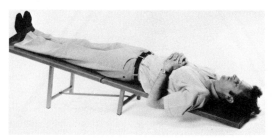

The **Gentle TIP-U-UP**:

★ Is portable, durable and light weight.
★ It stimulates circulation to all parts of the body – especially to the head. It helps relaxation, puts gravity to work for you, lifts sagging organs, helps your complexion, refreshes and invigorates your mind and body.
★ It may be used as an exercise board to help eliminate unwanted bulges, build the body where desired, tone the muscles and keep generally fit.

THE BACKSWING

The **Gentle TIP-U-UP** is 18″ high at the foot; however with the **BACKSWING**, the body can be varied in slant by shifting the centre of body weight and can be gently sloped or almost straight up and down. This separates the spinal discs and exercises them, so that after daily constant use, the spinal column can be relieved and many spinal problems alleviated – such as sclerosis, any type of curvature, slipped discs, pinched nerves, various muscle weaknesses and tension in ligaments, etc.

Inversion therapy – traction by hanging upside-down is a modern medical version of an ancient method of treating back problems. It is already attracting great interest among medical practitioners on both the orthodox and the 'alternative' side of the fence. In America, Britain and Europe, the

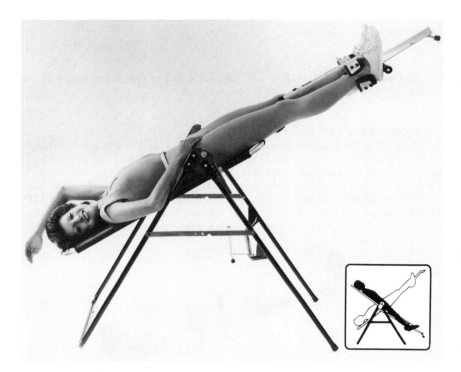

BACKSWING is being used in hospitals and clinics by sports doctors and orthopaedic specialists, as well as by individual patients and customers in their homes.

The method has been known since Hippocrates. Traction by inversion helps relieve the pressure on protruding intervertebral discs and compressed nerve roots, particularly in the case of low back pain. It improves the circulation of the blood and the drainage of the lymphatic system, it helps clear up static muscular fatigue, and may even clear blocked sinuses.

Use of the **BACKSWING** may not be advisable in some cases such as high blood pressure, and it is recommended that people with long-standing illnesses consult their doctors.

Because of the tremendous success of the **BACKSWING**, *there have been many attempts to produce an imitation machine.*

We do advise you to avoid such machines. *It is extremely unlikely that they will be of the same quality or as medically proven as the* **BACKSWING**.

Two models

The **Home Model** is neat, compact, sturdy and easy to use with uncomplicated instructions. Recommended for body weights up to 14½ stone (200 lbs). It requires a minimum 7' ceiling height and folds to 48″ × 26″ × 5″.

The **De-Luxe Heavy Duty Model** is suitable for clubs, clinics and hospitals. It takes body weight up to 20 stone (280 lbs).

50

CHAPTER NINE

BOWEL CLEANSING THROUGH THE USE OF ENEMAS

There is such emphasis in current fashion on external appearance, that usually the mere mention of the word *enema* invokes expressions of repulsion or embarrassment. The Yogis of old who maintained equilibrium between inner and outer cleanliness in a detached manner, always included enema techniques in their way of life. Their ancient texts, as well as the Essene Gospel, include information on methods of internal bowel cleansing. Originally, it is said, birds were observed to draw water into their beaks, insert their beaks into their rectum and then expel the water. Man then followed this example.

In modern times, the science of Iridology helps to prove the correlation of the colon to reflex disease, toxins and symptoms. Essentially, the colon is a hub: each segment of the bowel with its intricate multitudinous connections of circulation, lymph and nerves connect to specific reflex areas throughout the entire body. If one area of the colon is toxic, spastic or inflamed, the symptoms are not only found in the bowel itself, but also in the reflex area.

Also, in allopathic medicine – in surgery and autopsy – the poisonous toxic conditions that exist inside the bowel, which pollute the body via the bloodstream, can be viewed at first hand. The colon is supposed to serve as a reservoir from which the blood absorbs nutrients to circulate throughout the entire system. But when the colon is toxic, or impacted with faecal matter, poisons are distributed instead. Also the person is not satisfied by food, feels hungry and eats much more than he needs, because the nutrients are not absorbed and circulated.

In Dr. Bernard Jensen's excellent book: *Tissue Cleansing Through Bowel Management*, photographs clearly show the black toxic material which is eliminated during thorough bowel cleansing.

Often when a patient is asked if they are constipated, they immediately say, 'No'. On further discussion it is found that that may mean from one motion every day up to one every three days. This is considered normal by them. Does it follow that if you take in food three times or more a day, that you should eliminate only once a day or less? Children with relaxed healthy systems usually have about three movements per day. If you let food sit for three days, it deteriorates. Imagine how much more putrefactive it would become if it stays in the bowel for three days. Gas is manufactured and pressure causes further problems as the colon develops swellings and pockets which hold further deposits of toxic waste. Poisons from these toxic areas are carried throughout the entire system, causing toxaemia.

Almost every person needs bowel cleansing, and once the bowels are brought to clean normal activity, a regular maintenance program is advised. Just as a house requires spring cleaning and a car needs regular tune-ups, the bowel needs maintenance cleansing, so that toxic wastes do not build up.

Although complete bowel cleansing and maintenance requires herbs, diet, massage and often packs and poultices, enemas are a significant and useful aid which serve an important function in any bowel program. The various kinds of enemas and their suggested use are listed below:

How To Take An Enema

You will require the following:
1. A gravity flow enema bucket or bag, and
2. Two pints of enema fluid (various types listed below).

You will find your enema a simple and pleasant experience if you organize yourself well, set aside a relaxed half hour and provide yourself with something to do when you are retaining the enema (like radio, book, tapes, etc.)

Many people like to take their enema while they are soaking in a warm bath. Others prefer to do it on a rug on the floor, so they can go up into the Yoga shoulder stand or the plough posture. Others choose the use of a slant-board or TIP-U-UP, allowing gravity to aid retention. The main suggestion is for each person to find out what they like and then make it a dutiful function of health care. It helps to have a hook in a convenient place from which to hang the enema bag or bucket.

When you have everything together, lie down on your back, or on your right side, and press the lubricated tip of the enema tube into the rectum until it is firmly in place, using a little soap, vaseline or oil for lubrication. Release the tube lock and let the liquid begin to flow into the rectum. It is best to have the liquid at room temperature, as hot water will of course be uncomfortable and cold water is harder to retain. You can control the flow of the liquid with the tube lock if it begins to get uncomfortable. If the water hits a block of impacted faeces, you can stop the flow, massage the area, turn or go up into the shoulder stand until you feel ready to inject more. Ideally, you should be able to inject and retain for at least ten minutes, an entire quart of enema fluid. Sometimes the urge to release cannot be ignored and it is wise to let it go and begin all over again. As the bowel condition improves, it will be easier and easier to accept and retain all the liquid with a minimum of discomfort. As you want the liquid to flow up the descending colon across the transverse, and down the ascending colon, it is helpful to change positions and massage the area. Often when a strong urge to release comes, it usually lasts only for a minute or so, and if you breathe quickly, and/or turn your feet in circles at the ankle in both directions you can ride the storm and will find that the crisis passes. Remember – the more you need the positivity and help of the enema, the more your bowels will try to reject the enema fluid prematurely. Each time you do an enema, try to hold it longer than the time before. Stay lying on the right side or in the inverted posture. It is clearly necessary to recognize that once people experience the release of symptoms by the use of enemas, they may be tempted to overuse them, rather than master overeating or stricter aspects of habit change and body purification. Overuse of enemas can result in weakening of bowel tone, so it is important to realize when enemas should and should not be used.

The most important use of enemas is the service they add to any body purification program. Whenever any form of fasting or dietary regimen releases toxins into the blood and lymph, the enema is most effective in carrying away toxins out of the body. It is also a necessary part of any program dedicated to deep bowel cleansing. However, once the goal is achieved, the enema is used only on a maintenance basis, sometimes once a week and sometimes once a month, or whenever signs of impending colds or flu or digestive problems make themselves known. If the need for enemas is too often, the person should seek professional guidance, so that he does not weaken the system by overusing the enemas, also avoiding the cause of the congestion or problem.

Plain Water Enemas
A warm water enema will effectively cleanse the rectum and release toxins which may be causing headaches and flatulence. Its effects are superficial, but can be relied on whenever any of the other enema fluids are not readily available.

Herbal Enemas
Make a strong infusion of herbal teas or a decoction of roots and barks, strain and cool. Use 2 teaspoons of herb per pint of water, 4 tsp. for each quart. This may be made up in advance, but used preferably within 24 hours, though certain herbs keep up to 72 hours. However, once souring or scum appears, throw it away. It should be kept in a glass container in a fridge or cool place. Make herbal infusions or decoctions in stainless steel or enamelled pots only. Fuller details of all these herbs and other formulae can be found in *HERBS OF GRACE* by Farida Sharan.

Catnip	Mildly nervine, calming, soothing, relaxing. Effectively brings down fevers. Excellent for use with children.
Chamomile	Excellent for recuperative periods after illness or a healing crisis.
Detoxifying	Make a decoction of yellow dock and burdock roots, then add red clover and red raspberry infusions. Stimulates the liver to dump bile, thereby relieving stress and pain in a healing crisis.
Slippery Elm	Mucilagenous, soothing, softening and nourishing enema. Excellent to give if the patient is having trouble eating or retaining food, as the bowel absorbs the nutriment.
Sage	Warming, purifying.
Garlic Injection	Profoundly purifying, an excellent aid in the treatment of worms. Liquidize 4 cloves in 1 pt. warm water and strain.
Astringent	Witch hazel, bayberry, or white oak bark, used to help stop diahorrea and dysentery.
Flaxseed	Relieves inflammation, pain and bleeding (more effective if you add 2 tsp. liquid chlorophyll). Also aids healing process.
Wheatgrass Implant	Inject pure chlorophyll juice of wheatgrass which restores positivity to bowel and blood stream. Excellent for chronic dieases. Can be mixed 1:1 with rejuvelac (water from soaking wheat).

Coffee Enemas
The coffee enema is widely publicized these days as a part of cancer therapy and chronic care naturopathy. It is excellent to relieve healing crisis pain and discomfort, to stimulate the liver to dump bile by absorption of the coffee into the haemhorroidal veins and the portal vein, and to encourage deep cleansing of the colon by stimulating peristaltic activity. It is a regular part of the Gerson Therapy regimen and the Kelly cancer programme. The coffee enema is prepared by putting 3 tbsp. of drip ground coffee into 1 quart of distilled water

which has just been brought to the boil. Continue on the boil for 3 minutes and then simmer on very low heat for 20 minutes. Cool. Strain and inject while at body temperature. Retain 10–15 minutes. This can be done every morning when on a detoxification program or fast, and every hour during an acute healing crisis. The bowels continue to operate independently even when taking the coffee enema regularly and start functioning easily on their own after the coffee enema is discontinued. The coffee enema is recommended after a lymph massage to cleanse the colon of the lymph which has drained into the bowel, but not before sleep as it is too stimulating. A Herbal substitute for the coffee enema is: Red Clover, Yellow Dock root, Burdock and Red Raspberry.

Spirulina Enema
The use of spirulina plankton enemas together with fasting and purification programs is an excellent way to cleanse the colon and purify the blood stream as quickly as possible. Spirulina has the unique advantage of supplying strength and power through the absorption of the plankton into the bowel wall, as well as cleansing at the same time by softening the impacted faecal matter and stimulating peristalsis. Direct nutrition absorbed by the colon provides proteins and essential amino acids, laying a balanced foundation for easy purification, since hunger and weakness are prevented by the spirulina intake. The Spirulina Enema may be made as follows: Heat 1 blender full of distilled water to body temperature. Mix 2 tsp. spirulina powder with half a cup of cold water till you make a smooth paste. Add 2 tsp. glycerine (obtainable from the chemists) and stir together. Add this loose paste to a blender half full of the warm distilled water, and mix at slow speed. You can also use a whisk. Add the remaining distilled water slowly, to fill the blender. Fill the enema bag right away and use quickly.

This method will wash out the lower and upper bowel and encourage a complete peristaltic downward action. The plankton is also absorbed into the bowel wall, helping to soften, loosen and dilute the bowel contents. Inject the mixture a little at a time while lying on the right side. Move back and forth from left to right side, and massage the bowel area. If you feel that retention is impossible, then eject, and start the process over again. With practice the bowel becomes accustomed and eventually you will be able to retain a full enema of 2 quarts for 5–10 minutes, while massaging the abdomen. Use of the shoulder stand will help the spirulina to reach throughout the intestinal tract. The glycerine helps to emulsify the mixture, soften the impacted faeces and lubricate the walls of the colon. Take the enema the first night of any fast and for the next two nights. While you continue the fast, take one every other day and after the fast take once a month on a regular basis for effective bowel maintenance. Spirulina powder is better than grinding up tablets, being without additives.

Enema Equipment
There are a number of different types of enema kit available, the commonest being described herewith:

The **ENEMA/DOUCHE BUCKET** (A) is a non-brittle, white plastic, 1.2 litre (2 pint) capacity, 4.25″ diameter by 6.5″ high, bucket with gravity feed pvc tube, enema and douche nozzles, and tap. It has a hole on one flattened side to

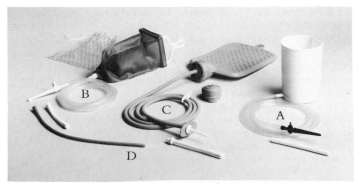

allow it to be hung on a wall-mounted hook and is easily cleaned from oils and strong herbs.

The **ENEMA/DOUCHE BAG** (B) is a strong, collapsible, 2 litre capacity, plastic bag with a reinforced top for mounting on a wall hook. It is easily cleaned inside. Packing into a small size, this enema kit is useful both for the home and when travelling, and comes complete with enema & douche nozzles and tap.

The **ENEMA/DOUCHE BAG** (C) is of the hot water bottle variety, with tube, clip, enema and douche nozzles, and a stopper for normal hot water bottle use. Useful for travelling as well as at home, but you can't get your hand inside if for cleaning. It is fine for warm water or well-strained herbal enemas.

There is also another variety, not pictured, sometimes called an **ENEMA SYRINGE**, which is simply a squeezable rubber bulb with a nozzle. They are useful for some applications, such as implants, but generally they do not hold enough fluid for a decent enema.

A useful addition for implanting the enema fluid higher up in the colon is a soft, flexible, 14″ **RECTAL IMPLANT TUBE** (D), with two laterally positioned end holes (rather than a single one in the end that gets blocked up). It fits all the enema kits, slipping over the standard rectal nozzle, also making insertion smoother and easier.

B. CASTOR OIL PACKS

Castor Oil Packs assist the enemas, because the absorption of the castor oil via the skin into the lymph system softens, relaxes, nourishes and balances the sympathetic and parasympathetic nervous systems when it is absorbed into the lacteals in the small intestine. It also disperses congestion and tension, and slowly helps to release the blockages in the bowel pockets. Dr. Christopher also comments, 'Castor Oil helps to get rid of hardened mucus in the body, which may appear as cysts, tumors, or polyps.' Many patients resist this treatment because they fear it will be messy. When they finally do it and are rewarded by the results, they always wish they had done it earlier.

Directions:

1. Over a plastic bin bag, place a cotton tea towel.
2. Soak the cotton cloth in castor oil.
3. Cover with second moist cotton cloth to provide heat.

4. Cover these two layers with plastic. Lift off the bottom plastic baggie and place over the abdomen.
5. Place a heating pad over this or use a hot water bottle (not so easy to manage, but it is not electric). Don't fill hot water bottles too full or they are too heavy.
6. Cover the entire lot with a thick towel which wraps around the body to hold everything in place. Secure by ties or pins.
7. Enjoy this soothing and relaxing pack for one and a half hours, 3 days in a row. Place the 2 layers of cotton and top layer of plastic back on the first layer of plastic, roll it up and put it away.
8. For the next 3 days massage the entire area with olive oil.
9. Rest on the seventh day, then repeat the entire procedure again.

Make sure you have organized yourself well to enjoy your castor oil pack. You can choose reading, writing, resting, meditating, T.V., conversation or even go to sleep. When I am tired, I let myself go to sleep and vaguely remember waking up, talking it off onto the plastic beside my bed and then going back to sleep. The relaxation of the solar plexus and abdominal emotional brain is very soothing and especially valuable to the kind of constipation caused by muscular tension.

One of the happy results of a clean colon is a more stable emotional life. It is said among natural healers that the constipated person is an irritable, impatient one. If we could only realize consciously the importance of internal hygiene on general health, well being and appearance, we would balance all our efforts for external appearance with internal cleanliness. It is certainly an essential aspect of any body cleansing program, whether for preventive or curative treatment. Once it is accepted into your life and has a place along with other beauty and health routines, you will be able to apply it when needed for beneficial results. Many people have a resistance towards accepting enemas and we hope this information will help you to overcome that. Your life will be the better for this knowledge.

CHAPTER TEN

IRIDOLOGY

Natural Diagnosis From The Iris Of The Eye

Iridology is the science of reading the signs – markings, structure and colourings – in the iris of the eye that reflect the state of health and basic constitution of the whole person, as well as the individual systems and organs. These markings reveal pathological and functional disturbances, and determine whether these imbalances are sub-acute, acute, chronic or degenerative. It is both an art and a science, requiring in its interpretation, logical, deductive skills and reasoning as well as intuitive wisdom, compassion and understanding. Every complex machine has an instrument panel to outwardly reflect its 'inward' condition. The iris is an extremely powerful and exact reflection of the state of the human body.

CHART TO IRIDOLOGY

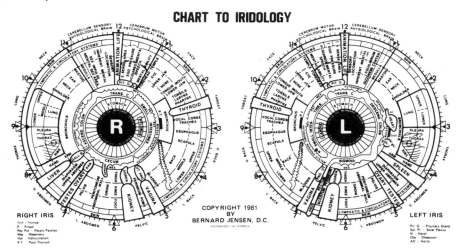

Courtesy Dr Bernard Jensen. Reprinted with Permission

The iris signs also show inherent weaknesses and whether crude, poisonous drugs or minerals have accumulated in the tissues. As well as pointing out the weak areas, iridology also shows where the strengths lie. Functional and organic changes are revealed long before they manifest as symptoms, and the body's strengths can be mobilized to throw off the accumulated toxins, and restore equilibrium of health.

Iridology is a common language, representing the inherent truth of this body we live in. It can be used efficiently and accurately with both allopathic and complementary medicine, as it is a diagnostic aid which complements other methods of diagnosis and integrates with any form of treatment. In Germany, it is utilized widely in surgery, for pinpointing exact areas for operations, especially in the gastro-intestinal tract. Several hundred medical doctors every year, take iridology training in a special school in the south of France. Even though the interest in England has come mostly from the complementary healing professions, there are wide possibilities for its use in orthodox medicine, as iridology offers inexpensive, safe, non-invasive and highly accurate methods of confirming diagnosis as well as monitoring the effects of treatment. In the U.S.A., Dr Jensen and others have pioneered this healing art, now using sophisticated, computerized image analysis to help identify iris markings. In Russia, doctors are using iridology in mental hospitals, where the information gained is used to guide cleansing and nutritional programmes, which when applied, relieve mental illness. The Soviet government has been very pleased, since patients can be discharged, thus saving the state large sums of money.

Used together with body purifying and regenerative therapeutic techniques and treatment, iridology shows living proof of natural healing – that suppression of disease is not a cure – and it provides a preventive approach to health as well as living warning of weaknesses developing in specific areas of the body. When the correct treatment is applied these markings change colour, develop healing lines or disappear altogether. The iris in health is bright, clean and clear, radiating the happiness of harmonious living.

A properly trained and qualified iridologist is a teacher who will guide his or her patients towards better health by involving them actively in their treatment. Iridology cannot exist separately from treatment. It is not enough just to read the iris signs and explain them to the patient. The information must be interpreted in terms of treatment to bring about tissue change and improvements in health. Students in iridology have come from all of the healing arts, including herbalists, homeopaths, acupuncturists, nutritionists, chiropractors, yoga teachers, osteopaths, kineseologists, medical doctors, ophthalmic opticians, nurses, physiotherapists, health food and wholefood shop owners, beauty therapy and health spa owners and directors, hypnotherapists, polarity therapists, naturopaths, reflexologists, vitamin therapists, etc. As a wholistic language, iridology serves to unite and bring practitioners of all the healing arts together in greater understanding.

We look outward into the world, using our eyes to interpret life in this world. When we turn our eyes inward, we begin to discover a deeper level of the reality of the life within us. Surely our achievements in this world will mean much more when we can enjoy a happier life with better health. Iridology is a useful tool to help us reach a more harmonious balance and a fuller life. We should not have to wait for our bodies to break down before we finally attend to health and try to repair what is left. An understanding of our body in both positive and negative aspects is essential for conscious responsible living. Iridology opens our eyes. Take a look. Healthier bodies will produce a healthier world.

In conjunction with the British School of Iridology, the Wholistic Research Company have developed and brought together a selection of equipment suitable for reading this human instrument panel.

To read the signs in the iris of the eye, the iris must be illuminated and magnified, hence one should use high quality pocket medical torches and good optical magnifiers. To make a permanent patient record, one can fill in a blank chart and ideally, take a photograph as well. For this purpose, we have designed our own **I-100 & I-800 IRIDOLOGY CAMERA SYSTEMS** with macro-light eye illumination, taking standard 35mm cameras, lenses and accessories.

Magnifiers and Torches

The use of cheap plastic magnifiers and torches should be avoided. 'Sherlock Holmes'-type magnifiers offer only a low magnification as well as introducing optical distortions which may even be unnoticed and read as iris signs. Pocket torches should be well constructed and use a lens-bulb to provide a small and focused, rather than diffused, light patch. Medical pocket torches are built to this specification, while household and map-reading torches are not. A mirror for reading your own iris is great fun, as well as being highly self-informative, and needs to create distortion-free magnification.

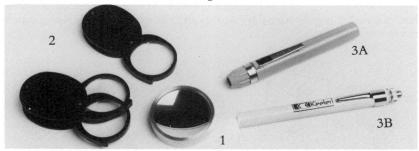

1. The **IRIDOLOGIST'S SELF-ANALYSIS MAGNIFYING MIRROR** gives a 6× magnification on a 1.5 inch diameter. The reflecting surface is optically ground, distortion-free and hardened, front-silvered. This mirror is our own design.
2. Amongst lenses we have found the **FOLDING POCKET MAGNIFIERS** to be the best. There is a 4×, 35mm diameter version and another with both 4× and 5× lenses, making 9× when used together. A minimum of 4× is essenial for iris readings.
3. There are two medical pocket torches we have found to be suitable. The **HEINE MINI-CLIPLAMP** (3A) is the more sturdily built, in an elegant grey, while the **KEELER MEDICAL PEN TORCH** (3B) has both a momentary (thumb operated), as well as a constant, light switch.
4. The **PEAK LIGHT LUPE**, with a 10× magnification, is the best torch plus magnifier combination we know. This model is recommended by Dorothy Hall in her book: *Iridology*.
5. The clarity and readability of iris markings is enhanced as much by stereo, 3-D (binocular) vision, as by simple magnification. When both eyes can be used, 4× magnification is all one needs, and the **STEREO HEADBAND**

4.

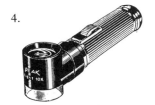

5.

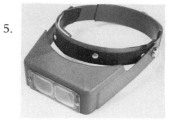

BINOCULAR MAGNIFIER provides a really good image of the iris – far better than a magnifier. It also leaves both hands free for note taking and holding a torch, which is also required.

Cameras

Taking notes and filling in a chart is a part of any iris diagnosis session. However, there is nothing like a photograph for an absolute record and reference. The condition and changes can be accurately recorded and discussed with patients on subsequent consultations using small table-top projection systems. Well documented and fascinating case-histories can also be compiled.

The Wholistic Research Company have devised two camera systems built around regular 35mm cameras with a 100mm (approx.) Macro Lens and appropriate extension bellows and/or rings. Special stands and modelling-plus-flash macro-lights have been designed specifically for iris photography and the results are very good.

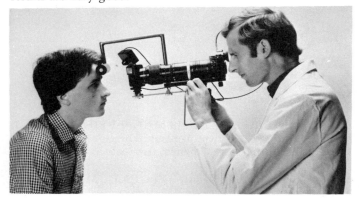

I-100
HAND-HELD

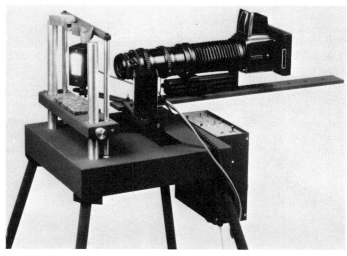

I-800

Iris Bioscopes

The iris of the eye is a wonderful structure. But until you have seen it *in full, stereo or three-dimensional, high magnification*, you have never really seen the iris. The depth of structures and their inter–relatedness take on a new dimension for you, quite unobtainable with simple lenses and magnifiers. Indeed, in West Germany, Josef Deck's school insists that all their students use Iris Bioscopes as essential instruments for diagnosis.

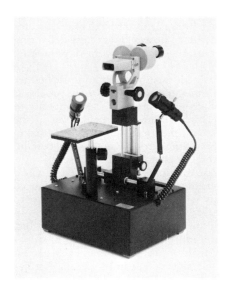

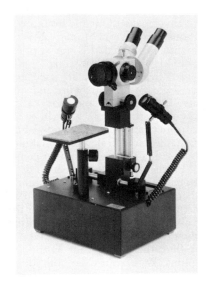

IB–240   IB–1000

Both the **IB–240** and **IB–1000** are designed to sit neatly across the corner of a table or desk, in order to take up absolutely minimum space. They are easy to use, portable and have been designed to give high magnification, stereo (3–D) viewing of the anterior chamber of the eye. The **IB–240** permits 10×, 20× and 30× magnifications, using separate lenses, while the **IB–1000** uses a more sophisticated stereo, iris bioscope head with a rotating lens system allowing instant changes of magnification from 4×, 6.3×, 10×, 16× & 25×.

CHAPTER ELEVEN

FURTHER MISCELLANEOUS ADJUNCTS TO A HEALTHY LIFESTYLE

Grain Mills, Herbal Tablet Makers, Heating Pads, Reflex Foot Rollers, Humane Mouse Traps, Stainless Steel Steamers, Aloe Vera Mother Plants

Grain Mills – Mill Your Own Additive Free Cereals And Pulses

Grains, pulses, flour and flour products have been a central part of man's diet for thousands of year. Modern agricultural methods, however, are now delivering grain and flour that is not as pure and natural as many modern-day thinking people would wish it to be.

Artificial fertilizers are used in practically all farming, while pesticides are used during both growing and storage of most grains. The ripening process is also foreshortened and modern strains of grain are bred for their response to chemical fertilizers, as well as for their high gluten content, useful in the commercial mass-production of bread. In fact, practically all the flour used in Britain's large-scale bread-making industry comes from Canada, not Britain, because of the higher gluten content in the Canadian wheat strains.

Furthermore, finely ground flours oxidise too quickly and we also eat wheat flour too often, due to availability, forgetting the other grains. In a balanced diet, variety can be the spice of life! Is it any wonder, therefore, that allergies to artificially grown grains are on the increase?

With organically-grown, additive-free flours being less readily available than the grains and pulses themselves, more and more people are turning to stone-milling their own flour as they need it, from verifiably, organically-grown grains. With your own mill you can be selective. You can buy grain that has been properly ripened from an organic farm growing an old breed.

You can avoid oxidation by fresh milling and using coarser grists. You can also give your body a change by using different grains. Rye, oats, maize, rice, millet and buckwheat, as well as pulses, lentils and chick-peas for example – can all be used to your nutritional advantage.

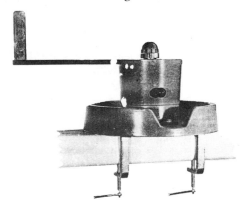

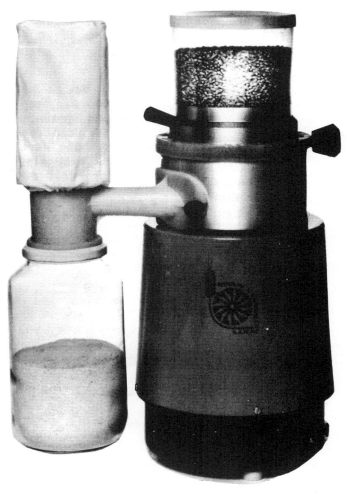

▲ B. The F-50 SAMAP Grain Mill

◀ A. The SAMAP Hand-Operated Grain Mill

The three **SAMAP** grain mills, available from the **Wholistic Research Company** are amongst the best we have found. They are stone-grinding, well-built and reliable. There is 12″ diameter **HANDMILL** (A), the **F-50** (B) motor-powered model with patented cooling turbine, which cools the grinding stones and the ground grain, preventing any heat build-up which would otherwise oxidize or de-nature the wheat-germ oil, vitamins and trace minerals and nutrients; and the **F-100** – a commercial model for bakeries, restaurants and communities. All three grain mills are adjustable to grind from coarse to very fine and the **F-50** and **F-100** have stackable hoppers so that you can leave the mill to get on with its work while you get on with yours.

Herbal Tablet Makers for the Home and Practice

The dispensing of herbs for personal consumption has long posed problems for patient and practitioner alike, as to how to take them without denaturing and reducing or altogether destroying their healing powers. Some herbalists prepare tinctures in alcohol, others use preparations from the large herbal pill companies, manufactured under pressure using industrial machinery. Those prescribing and dispensing dried herbs recommend herbal teas or the filling of gelatin capsules.

After some considerable experimentation into a variety of different methods of preparing herbal pills in comparatively small quantities for the home or practice, we came up with a simple and effective solution, (which we have patented), that totally replaces the time-consuming and dusty operation of filling gelatin capsules and may well induce herbalists to prescribe the dried herbs more readily. It is, of course, a matter of personal choice and experience, but it is good to have this alternative to capsules.

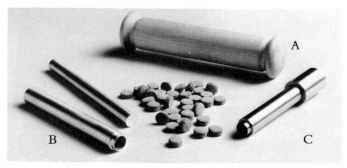

Firstly, the dried and powered herb is mixed with a firm, set honey. This is rolled out on a board, like pastry. The hand-turned, beechwood **TABLET ROLLER** (A) has rounded ends to provide a pestle for thorough mixing of the herb and honey. The ends are also of greater diameter than the roller surface, thus rolling the herb and honey mixture to a standard thickness. Using a little of the herb powder on the mixture, the roller and·the rolling board prevents sticking. The rolled out mixture is then cut into tablet shapes using a round stainless steel cutter, and the tablet is ejected using a stainless steel rod or ejector. In our **SIMPLE TABLET-MAKER** (B), the ejector is operated with a simple push while the **SPRING-LOADED TABLET-MAKER** (C) has a thumb-operated, spring-loaded ejector as an integral part of the cutter.

This tablet-making process has a number of distinct advantages over gelatin capsules:

1. Gelatin capsules are of animal origin and may be objectionable to vegetarians.
2. Honey has a natural resistance to bacterial and fungal attack and is a naturally occuring, nutritious food.
3. Making pills is several times faster than filling capsules, especially by hand.
4. Capsule filling creates a fine dust that can make you sneeze.
5. The recurring cost of gelatin capsules for even a short course of herbs is more than the once-only cost of a pill maker.

Heating Pads
Heat Therapy is as old as man and this modern 11″ × 15″ **Heating Pad** from Dreamland is a good one for use with herbal and castor oil packs or to give simple relief from muscular strains, aches and tensions.

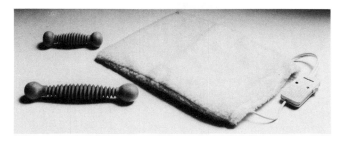

Reflex Foot Rollers
Like the eye in Iridology, or the ears in auricular acupuncture, the soles of the feet are an area of reflex energy and may be compared to a map of the whole body. They are covered in nerve endings and reflexes which correspond to the different organs. These reflex points have been accurately charted and used to promote healing in China and Tibet for hundreds of years, and more recently in the West.

Disturbance or disease in any organ or structure reflects in the feet as subtle energy disturbances in the area corresponding to the organ involved, slowing down circulation of blood and vital energy, or life force, to this organ. Clearing these (sometimes painful) spots or energy blockages by massage and stimulation, restores vitality, circulation and nerve supply to the effected organ, thus aiding its return to normal, healthy function.

REFLEX FOOT ROLLERS have been designed with this in mind. Used daily, the feet will normally become more supple. Circulation, for those who suffer from cold feet, should improve. Tender spots discovered by a foot roller and when worked upon, will begin to disappear. By studying the charts supplied with the roller, you can discover which organs correspond to your tender spots. For example, the shape of the arch reflects the shape of the spine.

Flat feet almost always indicate spinal problems, the symptom of which is back ache, if not in the present, then in the future. Working with a reflex foot roller and looking to your posture and breathing will help to rectify this.

There are two varieties:

The **MAXI REFLEX FOOT ROLLER** (10.5″ long by 1.5″ diameter) and the **MINI REFLEX FOOT** Roller (6″ long by 1.5″ diameter) are hand-turned in maple, beech or other suitable woods, and scented in aromatherapy sandalwood oil. They look good, feel good and also smell good.

Whole Live Mouse Traps – For the Betterment of Mousekind!

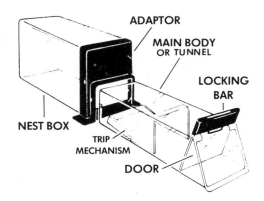

Maxi Trip-Trap – The Mini-Trap Has A Smaller Nest Box

With the drawing in of the cold autumn months, mice start looking for somewhere warm with a ready food supply to spend the winter and suddenly you find you have a mouse (or more) about the house. Every creature has a right to live and yet their presence is neither healthy nor safe (they can strip the PVC off electric cables). We have therefore found a humane mousetrap that really does work and allows you to release the mice easily (away from your home) without getting bitten.

Both the **MINI TRIP-TRAP** and the **MAXI TRIP-TRAP** catch one mouse at a time, without maiming or killing them. However, the **MAXI TRIP-TRAP** has enough space for food and bedding. Mice are sensitive to cold and hunger, so it helps them stay snug and well-fed until they can be released.

Trip-Traps are a completely new type of mousetrap. They are more hygenic and safer to use than conventional spring-traps and they cannot hurt children or domestic pets.

Stainless Steel Steamers
We imagine that most of our customers are already aware of the health hazards of aluminium cooking pans, as well as the advantages of steam cooking. Aluminium has been known for many years to be injurious to health. Recent

medical research shows that it disrupts nervous tissue function and is implicated in the development of senile dementia.

Cooking foods in a **STEAMER**, rather than boiling it, is obviously more beneficial, since the mineral and nutritional content is preserved intact, rather than being leached out and thrown away

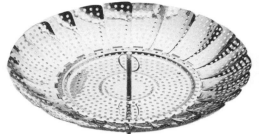

with the cooking water. Taste is also preserved too, and different vegetables can also be cooked alongside each other with minimal mixing of flavours.

Our folding, **STAINLESS STEEL STEAMERS** fit inside all saucepans and can also be lifted out and placed directly in a serving dish for ease and simplicity, helping to preserve both heat and flavour.

Aloe Vera *Mother Plants*

Though still little known in Europe, *Aloe vera* has long been prized on the American continent as one of nature's special healing plants, like comfrey and others. Says Michael Tierra in his well-loved book, *The Way of Herbs*, "The gel of the leaves of the aloe is most widely honoured for its capacity to heal even the most severe burns and irritated skin rashes, (this includes sunburn). In addition, it has been successfully applied for the treatment of insect bites and stings, poison oak and ivy, 'detergent hands,' acne and itchy skin. . . . As a first aid for burns and irritations, break off a leaf and squeeze the gel onto the affected area." The profuse gel of the *Aloe vera* provides healing substances and also dries to form a protective layer over any area of broken, irritated or inflamed skin. Used regularly on wounds, it also helps prevent the formation of scar tissue. Michael Tierra continues, "Taken internally, it is a laxative and regulator of the bowels. . . . Take the bitter aloe gel in small quantities at regular intervals . . . along with a tea of ginger and licorice root." The powerful healing properties of *Aloe vera* have also been used to advantage in the natural treatment of stomach ulcers and some forms of cancer – especially of the stomach and lung.

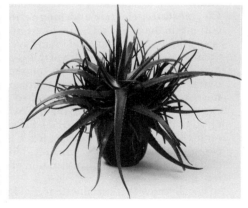

Aloe vera is a succulent that grows well in the home, rapidly reaching heights of 24 inches or more. But, most delightfully, each plant also becomes mother to a host of baby plants. Occasionally, a long and graceful flowering stem is also produced. As a first aid plant to grow in the house or office, there is nothing to equal it.

Our stock plants came originally from the Californian desert and though we have grown them to profusion in our own home, we have only recently put them into our list of products. We hope you will enjoy them as much as we have!

CHAPTER TWELVE

THE INDOOR ENVIRONMENT
VDU Filters, Full Spectrum Lighting, Allergy Control

Man's approach to the creation of his modern technological environment has largely been to go ahead with little understanding of the side-effects his activities will have upon his well-being and this is no more apparent than in the modern office. Space is at a premium – it costs money – as does maintaining it at a reasonable temperature etc., with the result that in the absence of a lack of understanding or perception of the subtle effects of the environment upon the humans involved, an ambience is created which induces stress, fatigue, headaches, apathy and worse, depending upon the reactions of the individual. The source of these problems is now becoming clear and solutions found, though vested interests may challenge the findings. We have identified products to balance air- ionization, to correct artificial lighting, to bring sunlight into a room even in mid- winter, to eliminate the electric fields around VDUs and to control environmental allergens such as dust mite.

Filters For Computer Terminals or VDU's (Visual Display Units)
Most VDU operators and those working with electrical equipment experience symptoms of tiredness and worse. Fatigue, of course, leads to loss of efficiency and mistakes. Many such workers take tiredness to be their lot, not realizing that it can have external causes that may be remedied. It is emotional, environmental and physiological stress (e.g. pollution or disharmony of all kinds) that can make one tired. Living one's day in a balanced frame of mind and in a natural environment will leave one fresh, not tired, as most of us experience when we go on holiday.
VDU operators suffer from:
1. **Glare** – due to incorrect lighting, reflections on the screen etc.
2. **Electrostatic, electric and magnetic field effects** create induced electric currents in the brain and body, interfering with their normal functioning. As is well-known, the body and brain have integral electrical activity as a part of their normal functioning. When this is even mildly disrupted, we experience it as "not feeling too good." Its long term effects may induce more serious illness as do other kinds of electromagnetic energy – X-rays, gamma rays, microwaves, radioactive decay and so on. You may perhaps have seen the experiment conducted on BBC TV where quite a large lump of gold was taped to the front of a TV set and left switched on for two years. When it was removed in front of the viewers, it had been converted to lead. The electrons zooming through the TV screen had induced radioactive decay and atomic change resulting in the disintegration of gold, with the ultimate formation of lead.

We all know that it is unsafe to sit right in front of our TV and yet this is exactly what VDU operators are asked to do, often for many hours per day. Electrons zooming through the brain, breaking up complex molecular structures and creating free radicals can hardly be considered harmless when one considers what they can do to the relatively simple atomic structure of gold. Free radicals are highly interactive bits of molecules that combine with anything around, breaking up the normal biochemical and electro-biological pathways.

The solution to glare and electrical problems lies in the use of **CONDUCTIVE ACRYLIC** or **MESH FILTERS.** Note that they must be **CONDUCTIVE**, the more readily available, non–conductive anti-glare filters solve less than half of the problems.

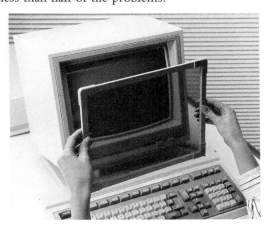

MESH FILTERS prevent glare by cutting out reflections. It is inexpensive, but can reduce resolution on high resolution displays, especially colour, where the colour dots (pixels) which comprise the screen can be obscured. This can be particularly marked at the edges. If the mesh is coated with an electrically conductive coating and if this is then connected to an electrical earth, then the electric field problems are also solved, *but not otherwise.*

ACRYLIC FILTERS are coated with an anti-reflection coating, thereby reducing glare. If the acrylic is also coated with a conducting material which is earthed, then the filter also removes the electric field problems, *but not otherwise.* The only drawback with acrylic is that under some extreme conditions (which can usually be remedied), there can be problems with reflection.

Generally speaking, the conductive acrylic filters are the best although they are a little more expensive.

The problems of providing a range of filters for a multitude of differently shaped VDU's also needs to be met and the **POWER SYSTEM VDU FILTERS** are the best range available. A badly fitting or badly positioned filter can be as bad or worse than the original.

Full Spectrum Lighting
Most offices are lit by normal fluorescent lighting which does not possess the combinations of wavelengths or colours found in natural sunlight. University and industrial researchers have reported on many occasions that the body absorbs light energy as a form of nourishment. This may seem like a new idea, but it is just what we are doing when we sunbathe, or just walk or sit outside.

And it is what plants do for a living. We may not be as good at it as they are, but it very definitely affects us.

Research reports show that humans, (as well as plants, chickens and pigs), all thrive when the lighting is changed to the full spectrum variety. Most lighting falls into two categories: fluorescent, and regular incandescent light bulbs.

For a domestic or office environment, we have unearthed the best daylight-mimicking, **INCANDESCENT LIGHT BULBS** in *bayonet* or *screw* fittings, and in using them have really noticed the difference. As have our house plants – some of them quite dramatically.

Normal incandescent light bulbs emit a light containing more red and yellow than natural daylight. The **PHILIPS DAYLIGHT BLUE** and **SUNGRO-LITE LIGHT BULBS** filter out this excess, providing a light that more closely approaches that of daylight. They were originally designed for use by painters, draughtsmen, printers and for applications where close colour matching or discrimination is critical, but have been found to be beneficial to human well-being and health. They enhance visual acuity and make reading easier. Office workers often find that they are less tired at the end of a day. They are also used extensively by plant growers because plants quite naturally get on better in light that more closely mimics the outdoor conditions. The **SUNGRO-LITE SPOTLIGHTS** are incandescent bulbs with a reflective base. This increases the effective light output and provides a more directional beam of light. Some folk prefer these for regular domestic or studio lighting.

Apart from the more general and positive effects upon health and well-being, the full or balanced spectrum emitted by these light bulbs and fluorescent tubes is used extensively by doctors, designers, painters and draughtsmen, etc. Colours are more sharply defined, as are details. Normal light bulbs and fluorescent tubes emit a yellowish light which blends colours and lends a slight fuzziness to whatever you are reading, examining or working upon. Using full spectrum lighting, however, visual acuity or sharpness of vision is improved, making work less tiring, and many folk find that they can even read more easily without their glasses.

We have installed full spectrum lighting in our home and office and feel very pleased with the results. We never previously realized how YELLOW is the light from normal artificial lighting, and what it does to one's perception of the environment.

The SUNBOX – Mount A Sunny Window on Your Wall!

Sunlight is essential to health and well-being, and in some instances, sunlight deprivation – as in winter – can induce a form of depression, known as SAD or Seasonal Affective Disorder. SAD is an acute form of winter lethargy or tiredness – the winter blues – that many of us suffer from during the winter. This winter depression is often accompanied by weight gain and can affect domestic and professional life. Some people also find that they require as much as four hours extra sleep. Symptoms differ with individuals, but the seasonal nature of the depression is usually obvious to most sufferers.

There is a physiological basis for SAD, involving the nervous and endocrine systems. The full details are not fully understood, but it is known that there are nervous and endocrine centres in the brain and body which closely affect our moods. The amount of light falling on the retina of the eye influences one – and possibly more – of these centres, which in turn affects the pineal gland, modifying the amount of the hormone *melatonin*, which it secretes.

Melatonin is a hormone of the brain and nervous system, circulating throughout the body, and involved in a variety of functions including mood and emotional balance. Basically – through the melatonin connection – sunlight makes you feel good and an absence of it can make you feel awful.

The solution to SAD is very simple: daily exposure to bright light greatly alleviates or even completely cures the symptoms. But the light needs to be *bright*, medical experiments determining that a brightness of 2,500 lux is about right. This is roughly the same brightness as experienced while standing at a window, surveying a sunny scene. By comparison, ordinary indoor lighting is usually no more than 200–500 lux, while a Mediterranean beach at midday is about 100,000 lux.

The **SUNBOX** was designed to provide diffuse and comfortable lighting of 2,500 lux at a distance of one metre (about 3 feet). The unit measures 920 x 630 x 85 mm (36″ × 25″ × 3½″), weighs 19kg, and is designed to hang on the wall, giving the effect of a four-paned cottage window. Treatment involves sitting about 3 feet away from the **SUNBOX** and doing whatever you want to do. Reading, study-ing, knitting, cooking, writing, sewing, eating and so on, are all activities that can be carried out during light therapy.

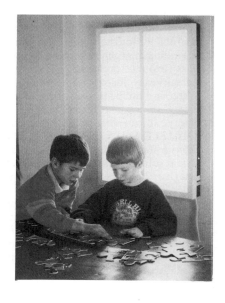

About 2 to 4 hours of daily exposure to bright lights have been shown to be necessary for effective treatment, depending upon the person. Marked im-provement in one's condition should be noticed within a week of starting treatment, but will recur within 3 days once treat-ment is stopped. For some reason, light therapy is most effective in the mornings and patients are en-couraged to use the **SUNBOX** between 7 and 9 a.m., if possible, though light therapy is effective until early evening. There are, of course, no adverse side effects, though looking directly into the light for long periods should be avoided. The **SUNBOX** does not cause tanning as no ultra-violet light passes through the diffuser.

Allergy Control in the Home

There are many forms of allergy, but in pursuit of a healthy indoor environment, we have concentrated on the single most common domestic source of allergic symptoms: house dust. And though there are many constituents of house dust to which people can be allergic, the commonest of all is the dust mite.

Dust mites are microscopic, insect-like creatures that inhabit all our homes, thriving in warm and humid conditions, living on a diet of shed, human skin scales. Mattresses, pillows, woollen blankets, carpets, unholstered furniture and all domestic fabrics, make ideal homes for them. But of them all, the warmth, humidity and regular replenishment of food, make mattresses, pillows and bed linen their most favoured habitat.

Female mites lay 25 to 50 eggs and – with a life cycle lasting only three weeks – it is easy to see how their numbers can rapidly increase to tens of thousands. Mattresses can contain exceptionally large numbers of dust mites – both dead and alive – and it is the excreta of these mites to which so many people are allergic.

Asthma studies indicate that not only can attacks be brought on by the dust mite, but that exposure to the dust mite can be one of the major factors contributing to the onset of asthma in children. Similarly, eczema, rhinitis and other allergic conditions can all be induced or made worse by the dust mite.

Fortunately, there are a number of effective measures which can be taken to control house dust and the house dust mite. And because we spend one third of our life in bed, the bedroom is the first place to start.

1. Use **DUST-PROOF MATTRESS, PILLOW AND DUVET COVERINGS**. The **Allergy Control** coverings we offer are made from a cotton–polyester blend fabric, laminated on the inside with a dust-proof coating. Once the mattress or pillow is encased in one of these covers, the offending allergen cannot escape into the environment and skin scales cannot pass through, depriving the mite of its food. A full, gussetted end-zipper permits easy dust-proof insertion, and encasings are machine washable in hot water and can be tumble-dried at low heat. All covers are also guaranteed for five years against defects in workmanship and materials.

2. Spray all carpets, mattresses, upholstery and soft furnishings with a **DILUTE SOLUTION OF TANNIC ACID**, which denatures allergens from mites, pollen, feathers and animal dander, rendering them harmless. The results of this treatment – which lasts 3 to 6 months – can be observed in less than 24 hours. Tannic acid is a natural compound, found in many trees as a natural defence against attacking organisms and insects. Unlike a number of other anti-allergy sprays, the spray contains no toxic chemicals, such as *benzyl derivatives*, which can accumulate in the body.

3. One of the major sources of *atmospheric* dust is your vacuum cleaner, most of which are so poorly filtered that dust is blown out from all the joints, as well as through the outlet filter. The characteristic smell of vacuum cleaning is actually the smell of dust particles – some of which can be severly allergenic. There are two ways of handling this problem. Either, you can fit your conventional vacuum cleaner with a special **VACU-FILT ALLERGY CONTROL VACUUM EXHAUST FILTER** or you can purchase a special vacuum cleaner. And the best of these, according to all the scientific tests, is the **MEDIVAC**.